Parasites and Pets: A Veterinary Nursing Guide

Hany M. Elsheikha, *BVSc, MSc, PhD, FRSPH, PGCHE, FHEA, DipEVPC*

University of Nottingham

Ian Wright, *BVS, MSc, MRCVS*

Mount Veterinary Practice

John McGarry, *MSc, PhD, SFHEA*

University of Liverpool

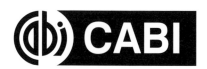

CABI is a trading name of CAB International

CABI
Nosworthy Way
Wallingford
Oxfordshire OX10 8DE
UK

CABI
745 Atlantic Avenue
8th Floor
Boston, MA 02111
USA

Tel: +44 (0)1491 832111
Fax: +44 (0)1491 833508
E-mail: info@cabi.org
Website: www.cabi.org

Tel: +1 (617)682-9015
E-mail: cabi-nao@cabi.org

A catalogue record for this book is available from the British Library, London, UK.

Library of Congress Cataloging-in-Publication Data

Names: Elsheikha, Hany, author. | Wright, Ian M., author. | McGarry, John W.,
  author. | C.A.B. International, issuing body.
Title: Parasites and pets : a veterinary nursing guide / Hany M. Elsheikha,
  Ian Wright, John McGarry.
Description: Wallingford, Oxfordshire ; Boston, MA : CABI, [2018] | Includes
  bibliographical references and index.
Identifiers: LCCN 2017040051 (print) | LCCN 2017055498 (ebook) | ISBN
  9781786394057 (ePDF) | ISBN 9781786394064 (ePub) | ISBN 9781786394040
  (pbk. : alk. paper)
Subjects: LCSH: Domestic animals--Parasites. | Veterinary parasitology. |
  MESH: Parasitic Diseases, Animal--nursing | Pets--parasitology | Animal
  Technicians | Examination Questions
Classification: LCC SF810.A3 (ebook) | LCC SF810.A3 E47 2018 (print) | NLM
  SF 810.A3 | DDC 636.089/696--dc23
LC record available at https://lccn.loc.gov/2017040051

ISBN-13: 978 178639 404 0 (paperback)

Commissioning editor: Jill Northcott
Editorial assistant: Emma McCann
Production editor: James Bishop

Typeset by SPi, Pondicherry, India
Printed and bound in the UK by Bell and Bain Ltd, Glasgow

Contents

About the Authors

Hany M. Elsheikha, BVSc, MSc, PhD, FRSPH, PGCHE, FHEA, DipEVPC

Hany is an Associate Professor of Veterinary Parasitology at the School of Veterinary Medicine and Science, University of Nottingham. He earned his PhD in Molecular and Evolutionary Parasitology from Michigan State University, where he studied the genetic population structure of the protozoan *Sarcocystis neurona*, the agent of equine protozoal myeloencephalitis in the Americas. In 2005, he was awarded the National Center for Infectious Diseases (NCID), Centers for Disease Control and Prevention (CDC) Postdoctoral Fellowship. He is the author of more than 250 research and professional articles on parasite pathobiology and control. Hany is the author of one US patent and three textbooks. Also, he is a diplomate of the European Veterinary Parasitology College (EVPC), a member of the European Scientific Counsel of Companion Animal Parasites (ESCCAP) UK & Ireland, a Fellow of the Royal Society of Public Health (RSPH) and a Fellow of the Higher Education Academy (HEA). From 2014 to 2015, Hany was the inaugural Specialty Chief Editor of Parasitology in the journal *Frontiers in Veterinary Science*. He serves on the Editorial Board of five peer-reviewed journals and as Reviewer of several journals and national and international funding agencies. Since 2007 he has been at the University of Nottingham, where he established the veterinary parasitology curriculum from its inception. Hany is also a veterinarian by training; he obtained a first-class degree with distinction in Veterinary Sciences and MSc in Veterinary Parasitology from Cairo University. His research focuses on host–parasite interaction and anti-parasitic drug discovery.

Ian Wright, BVS, MSc, MRCVS

Ian is a practising veterinary surgeon and co-owner of the Mount Veterinary Practice in Fleetwood, Lancashire. He has a Master's degree in Veterinary Parasitology, is head of the European Scientific Counsel of Companion

Animal Parasites (ESCCAP) UK & Ireland and guideline director for ESCCAP Europe. Ian has regularly published in peer review journals and is an editorial board member for the *Companion Animal* journal as well as peer reviewing for journals such as *Journal of Small Animal Practice* (JSAP), *Companion Animal* and *Veterinary Parasitology*. He continues to carry out research in practice, including work on intestinal nematodes and tick-borne diseases.

John McGarry MSc, PhD, SFHEA

John is a Senior Lecturer in Parasitology. He completed his PhD on vector ecology in 1992, at the Liverpool School of Tropical Medicine where he worked for 28 years and completed numerous projects in Africa. He has worked at the Institute of Veterinary Science since 2008. Research interests are the biology and control of parasitic arthropods – principally flies, ticks and mites – as agents of skin infestations and vectors of disease; more recent interests are parasitic lungworms of companion animals, zoonotic helminths of wildlife and forensic entomology, a pathology-related veterinary specialism. He is the author of some 70 publications of international repute.

Preface

This parasitology book is first and foremost designed for the veterinary nurse – the profession's most valuable asset. Dogs and cats frequently encounter a diverse variety of internal and external parasites; some cause mild symptoms in the pet, others are life threatening, and in some cases human health may be at risk too. Some parasites are very common indeed, such as the roundworm *Toxocara canis*, and fortunately can be easily and effectively controlled; others, such as certain tick-borne pathogens, may occur sporadically, for example during pet travel, and being perhaps unfamiliar, present a real diagnostic and management challenge for the nurse and practitioner. Nurses are at the very front of the clients' questions and are asked an astonishing amount about infections and parasites, a familiar enquiry being, 'Can I catch this from my dog?' With the nurse in mind, there has long been a need for a reference book that answers such questions posed in this format and which describes common parasites of cats and dogs, the diseases they cause, treatment options and prophylactic measures.

The subject matter of this book focuses primarily on parasitic diseases of dogs and cats in Europe and North America, but many of these are of course a global problem and the information herein is therefore suitable for a wide veterinary audience. The book format is designed for quick reference and will provide essential practical knowledge and training necessary in supporting veterinary surgeons and in providing concise information to clients. The book is composed of ten chapters. Chapter 1 gives a brief overview of parasitology; the following six chapters describe specific parasite problems encountered in small animal practices, and the final three chapters are dedicated to principles of parasite diagnostics and control. Self-assessment questions, answers to which can be found at the end of the book, are formative, to test the reader's understanding of major topics of parasite life cycles and therapeutics.

Therapeutics is an ever-changing field. Readers of this book are advised to check the most up-to-date product information provided by the manufacturer of each drug to verify the recommended dose, the method and duration of administration and adverse effects. It is the responsibility of attending veterinary professionals to be familiar with the laws governing drugs in their practice areas. Neither the publisher nor the authors assume any liability for any injury and/or damage to persons or property with the use of material(s) and information contained in this book. The mention of trade names or commercial products in this book is solely for the purpose of specific information and does not imply recommendation or endorsement by the publisher or authors.

The book is dedicated to veterinary nurses, students and practitioners. We hope you find this a very useful resource.

Hany M. Elsheikha
Ian Wright
John McGarry

1 Introduction to Parasitology

What is parasitology?

Parasitology is the scientific discipline concerning the study of the biology of parasites and parasitic diseases. By understanding parasites, their behaviour and life cycles, it becomes possible to develop strategies to treat and control parasitic disease.

What is a parasite?

A parasite is an organism that is metabolically and physiologically dependent on another organism (the host). The parasite exploits the host for its development and survival during one or more stages of its life cycle. Some parasites are single-celled (e.g. protozoa) whereas others are multicellular (e.g. worms, arthropods). In many cases, two (or more) parasites can occur in the same host and this phenomenon is known as poly- or hyper-parasitism and the host is said to be co-infected.

How does a parasite get its name?

Scientific nomenclature assigns each parasite two names; the genus name is the first name and the first letter is always capitalized, followed by species name (e.g. *Ixodes ricinus*) (Fig. 1.1). By convention, both names are italicized. Normally, after a scientific name has been mentioned once, it is abbreviated with the initial of the genus followed by the species name.

How did the names of parasites originate?

Veterinary professionals and parasitologists must become familiar with both the scientific (i.e. the classification according to Linnaean taxonomy) and common names of parasites (e.g. *Toxocara canis*, the dog roundworm). Many parasite species have a preferred site of final development (i.e. site of predilection) within the host body. In many cases, the organ of preference

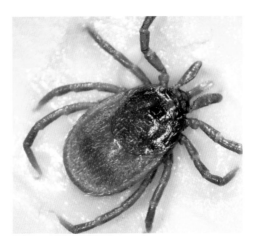

Fig. 1.1. Dorsal view of *Ixodes ricinus*. Also known as the sheep tick, wood tick, or deer tick.

provides the common name for the parasite. Examples are the 'eyeworm' (*Thelazia*) and the 'heartworm' (*Dirofilaria immitis*). Some worm species received a common name from their distinctive body shape, such as nematodes of genus *Trichuris*, known as 'whip worms', due to their characteristic whip-like shape. Likewise, the intestinal nematodes of dogs and cats, *Ancylostoma* spp. and *Uncinaria stenocephala*, are commonly known as 'hookworms'.

How big are the parasites?

Parasites range in size from tiny protozoa a few microns in diameter (little more than the size of some bacteria) to very large indeed; for example, the *Taenia* species tapeworms of dogs can measure several metres in length.

What are the major taxonomic groups of parasites?

In this book we shall cover common parasites in the taxonomic groups: Nematoda (roundworms), Cestoda (tapeworms), Trematoda (flatworms), Arthropoda (insects, acarines) and Protozoa. Nematodes, cestodes and trematodes are collectively known as helminths (worms).

What are the differences between ectoparasites and endoparasites?

Parasites can be divided as above based on sites they infect or infest. Ectoparasites are external and feed or live on the body surface of the host. They may suck the blood (Fig. 1.2) and lymph or feed upon feather, hair, skin and its secretions. Most ectoparasites are arthropods, i.e. invertebrates with jointed legs and hard external skeletons, e.g. lice, ticks, mites, fleas, bugs, flies, and mosquitoes. Endoparasites are internal (i.e. they live inside the host), such as worms (Fig. 1.3) that live in the gut, tissues or other organs.

2 Parasites of the Gastrointestinal System

Ascariasis of Dogs and Cats

What is ascariasis of cats and dogs?

Ascarid infections of dogs and cats are cosmopolitan. Adult worms live in the small intestine of dogs (*Toxocara canis* (Fig. 2.1a) and *Toxascaris leonina*) or cats (*Toxocara cati* (Fig. 2.1b) and *Toxascaris leonina*). Fertilized females produce eggs that become infective in the environment after being passed in faeces. Infections are well tolerated in cats and dogs but can lead to ill thrift and respiratory signs in heavily infected individuals, typically puppies and kittens. Pathology associated with ascarid infections in dogs and cats involves inflammatory and pathological alterations in the intestinal mucosa (caused by adults) and hepatopulmonary tissues (caused by migrating larvae).

What happens after a dog ingests T. canis *eggs?*

After a dog eats viable, embryonated eggs (Fig. 2.2) from the environment, the eggs hatch and escaped larvae enter the wall of the small intestine. The larvae migrate through the circulatory system and go to either the respiratory system or other organs/tissues in the body. If they enter body tissues, they encyst, especially in older dogs and pregnant bitches. In very young puppies, larvae move from the circulation to the respiratory system, are coughed up and swallowed and mature into adult worms in the small intestine. These adult worms lay eggs, which pass out of the animal in the faeces 4–5 weeks post infection and mature in the environment within 2 weeks to several months, depending on the soil type and environmental conditions such as temperature and humidity. Eggs become infectious and can remain viable for at least 1 year under optimal circumstances.

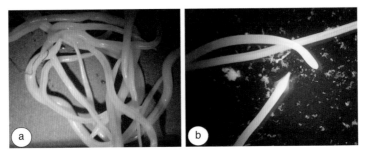

Fig. 2.1. Roundworms of dogs and cats. (a) Adult *Toxocara canis*, the most common intestinal roundworm of dogs. (b) Adult *Toxocara cati*, the most common intestinal roundworm of cats.

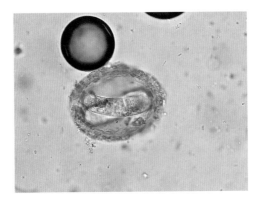

Fig. 2.2. Larvated egg of the dog roundworm, *Toxocara canis*.

What are the clinical signs of dogs infected with Toxocara?

Low-intensity infection does not cause signs of disease. Young puppies and kittens are most likely to show clinical signs and these will be worse if they have a large number of worms or migrating larvae. Signs include coughing, nasal discharges, vomiting, diarrhoea, stunted growth rate, distended abdomen (pot-bellied appearance), or pale mucous membranes. Death is rare, but has been reported and has been due to obstruction of the intestine or ulceration and perforation of the intestine wall.

Do paratenic hosts have a role in Toxocara transmission?

If a cat or dog eats a paratenic host (see Glossary for definition), any encysted larvae present will migrate in the animal in a way similar to that if infective eggs had been ingested. This route of infection is of particular importance in hunting cats preying on mice with *Toxocara* larvae in the tissues.

Tranplacental transmission is another route for T. canis. *How does it occur in the bitch?*

The dormant larvae in the tissues of a pregnant bitch can migrate through the uterus and placenta and infect the fetal puppy. This is called in-utero-transplacental transmission. The intrauterine infection is the most important mode of transmission in puppies, with close to 100% of puppies being infected, resulting in egg excretion by the puppy after a minimum period of 16 days.

Can puppies get infected with T. canis *via milk?*

Yes, larvae can also enter the female's mammary tissues. The puppies can become infected through the milk while nursing. The swallowed larvae mature in the puppy's intestine. Larvae have been found to pass in the bitch's milk for at least 5 weeks post partum.

What are the routes to T. cati *transmission in cats?*

In cats, transmission occurs by three mechanisms: (i) ingestion of eggs; (ii) ingestion of larvae in paratenic hosts; and (iii) transmammary transmission. Transmammary passage of larvae occurs in the colostrum and throughout the first 3 weeks of lactation. This mode of transmission is the most important source of infection in kittens. Unlike *T. canis*, prenatal infection via the placenta does not occur with *T. cati*.

Does Toxocara *infection have a public health impact?*

Very much so. *Toxocara* roundworms of dogs and cats have significant public health implications. Humans are infected by the accidental ingestion of infective embryonated *Toxocara* eggs present in contaminated soil (geophagia), dog hair, unwashed hands or raw vegetables. Untreated puppies are a major source of environmental contamination, as they can excrete millions of *Toxocara* eggs in a day. Infection can also occur through the consumption of undercooked game and offal but this thought to be uncommon. The larvae hatch from the ingested eggs, penetrate the small intestine and migrate to different tissues in the body, inducing inflammatory responses. Migration of *Toxocara* larvae leads to a number of syndromes, including visceral larva migrans (VLM), ocular larval migrans (OLM), neurological toxocariasis (NT) and covert toxocariasis (CT). The severity of symptoms depends on the number of infective eggs ingested. Risk of disease in humans is particularly high in: (i) children with pica tendency (i.e. soil-eating), because they are more likely to ingest embryonated eggs from soil and contaminated items than those not exhibiting this behaviour; (ii) children between 2 and 4 years of age; and (iii) individuals growing up in a poor socio-economic area. *T. leonina* is increasingly thought to have some zoonotic potential but is of less importance than the risk from *T. canis* and *T. cati*.

Can pet owners become infected via contact with their dog's fur?

The fur of dogs has been demonstrated to be a source of *T. canis* eggs for human infection. However, contact with pets harbouring patent *T. canis* infection is usually not considered to be as high a risk as ingesting soil, pica and sand contamination. This may be because the rate of successful embryonation in fur is not as high as in soil, but there is still a potential risk for infection from this route and good hand hygiene is always advisable after contact with dogs.

How do you diagnose toxocariasis in dogs and cats?

Toxocariasis in dogs and cats is diagnosed primarily on the basis of clinical criteria during examination. In large numbers, the parasite causes diarrhoea, emesis, stunted growth, abdominal discomfort and, in severe cases, intestinal obstruction and distended abdomen (pot-bellied appearance). Laboratory diagnosis of patent *Toxocara* infections is achieved by the detection and specific identification of *Toxocara* eggs in the faeces, following a concentration technique. *Toxocara* eggs are rough-shelled, spherical or oval and approximately 87 × 75 μm (*T. canis*) (Fig. 2.3) and 75 × 65 μm (*T. cati*).

Concentration/flotation techniques, however, are insensitive and may miss up to one-third of patent infections, not least because shedding of eggs may occur intermittently. The development of rapid, highly sensitive and specific diagnostic tests that can be executed in the field is an essential element in any future control programmes. Faecal antigen testing is one such example and is becoming commercially available. This will provide a sensitive and

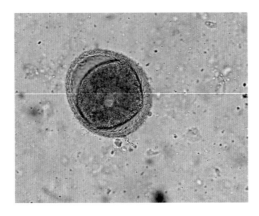

Fig. 2.3. *Toxocara canis* egg. Note the pitted appearance of the surface of the egg shell.

specific alternative to faecal flotation/concentration of eggs (see Chapter 8) but will not detect immature adults in the gut or be able to detect arrested larval stages in the tissues.

What is the current position for human toxocariasis in the UK?

Clinical human toxocariasis seems to be uncommon in England and Wales with approximately two cases per million people per year reported to the Health Protection Agency (HPA) Centre of Infections each year. This is likely to be a gross underestimate, as UK seroprevalance is approximately 2%. Diagnosis is complex, since signs are non-specific and vague, similar to other infections and thus easily misdiagnosed. The disease is not notifiable and source of the data is based on voluntary reporting by microbiology laboratories.

What are the recommended control measures for toxocariasis and best practice for public health?

Puppies and kittens provide by far the largest source of potential infection. Treatment of puppies should start at 2 weeks of age, repeated at 2-weekly intervals until 2 weeks post weaning and then monthly until 6 months old. This is to eliminate *T. canis* egg shedding from transplacental and trans-mammary infection and significant populations establishing in the intestine. Kittens should be treated in the same way but the first treatment can be given at 3 weeks old as there is no transplacental transmission. Nursing bitches and queens should be treated concurrently with their offspring, since they may develop patent infections. It has been demonstrated that use of an effective anthelmintic every 3 months significantly reduces *Toxocara* spp. egg shedding and there is no evidence that less frequent deworming will have any effect on egg output over time. Therefore, deworming every 3 months should be a minimum recommendation in dogs and cats unless frequent faecal testing for ova or antigen is being performed. Use of a monthly anthelmintic will significantly reduce egg output and whether this is necessary will depend on the pet's life style. Those pets hunting, in contact with young children, immunosuppressed individuals or individuals with poor hygiene should be dewormed monthly. However, it should be remembered that anthelmintics at the normal doses are not effective against encysted somatic larvae and subsequent shedding of eggs may occur if routine treatments are not maintained.

Since no effective or practical methods exist for reducing existing environmental egg contamination, prevention of contamination build-up in the environment and good hygiene and practice are the key points in the prevention of toxocariasis. In practice, measures should be focused on the following four principal points.

11

1. Regular deworming of cats and dogs.

2. Limiting access of dogs and cats to public areas, especially those frequented by small children, such as playgrounds.

3. Education of pet owners to cover sandpits to prevent cat defecation when not in use, prevent defecation of pets in public areas and clean up faeces from soil and on pavements. Local authorities have implemented a variety of interventions to tackle dog fouling, including placing notices in public areas, leaflet distribution, enforcement, media coverage, provision of free 'poop scoops', convenient placement of dog waste bins, fines and DNA testing of dog faeces to identify ownership.

4. Good hygiene, including regular hand washing and thorough washing of fruit and vegetables intended for human consumption.

Public awareness is essential for the control and prevention of human toxocariasis. Pet owners' lack of understanding of parasites and their zoonotic implications underpin many of the potential public health problems currently faced. Uniform guidelines for the control and treatment of parasites in pet animals have been developed and published by the Companion Animal Parasite Council (CAPC) in the USA (www.capcvet.org) and the European Scientific Counsel for Companion Animal Parasites (ESCCAP) in Europe (www.esccap.org). These guidelines provide an overview on different worm species and their clinical and zoonotic significance, and enable pet owners and veterinarians to make informed decisions on the selection of rational control measures in order to mitigate the risk of *Toxocara* infection.

What drugs are available to treat T. canis *infection in dogs?*

A wide assortment of drugs is available for use against *T. canis*. These include benzimadazoles (e.g. fenbendazole, mebendazole), macrocyclic lactones (MLs) (e.g. milbemycin, moxidectin), tetrahydropyrimidines (e.g. pyrantel pamoate) and octadepsipeptides (e.g. emodepside). Because pregnant and nursing bitches are sources of infection, they should be treated after whelping. Fenbendazole has been shown to reduce transmammary and transplacental transmission if given every day from day 40 of pregnancy to 2 days post parturition.

How do you treat and control T. cati *infection?*

Treatment and control of *T. cati* is very similar to *T. canis*, with *T. cati* being susceptible to a similar range of anthelmintics and with zoonotic transmission occurring by the same routes. Feral and stray cats significantly contribute to *Toxocara* egg contamination of the environment. Cats will also defecate and bury their faeces in high-risk areas for people, such as allotments, sandpits and children's play areas. It is important, therefore, to

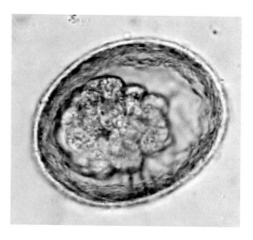

Fig. 2.4. Egg of the dog and cat roundworm *Toxascaris leonina*.

consider stray cat control when looking at control programmes for human toxocariasis as well as ensuring that sandpits are covered when not in use.

What are the clinical signs of dogs infected with Toxascaris leonina?

They are similar to those for *T. canis*.

How is T. leonina *transmitted?*

Transmission occurs via two routes.

1. Through ingestion of infective eggs. The eggs hatch and the larvae mature within the small intestine, becoming adult females which pass eggs in the faeces and hence into the environment, where they develop.
2. Through ingestion of larvae in a transport or intermediate host, mainly mice and other rodents.

The prepatent period for *T. leonina* is about 11 weeks.

How do you diagnose, treat and control T. leonina?

The egg surface of *T. leonina* (Fig. 2.4) is smooth. This characteristic is used to differentiate between *T. leonina* and *Toxocara* species. For diagnosis, flotation methods are used to concentrate eggs from faeces (see Chapter 8). Treatment and control are similar to *T. canis*.

Hookworm Infection

Like ascarids, these too are common worms of dogs and cats and are also found in the small intestine and produce eggs, which can be found in faeces. The eggs look rather different to ascarid eggs, however.

How do hookworms get their name?

The name is derived from the head end being bent dorsally to create a 'hook' shape to the front end of the parasite. Of note are the mouths of hookworms – a large cavity (the buccal capsule) which in the case of *Ancylostoma caninum* (in dogs) and *Ancylostoma tubaeforme* (in cats) has three pairs of sharp teeth at the ventral rim, while *Uncinaria stenocephala* (in dogs) lacks these teeth and the margin is instead armed with rounded plates. *A. caninum* females measure 15–18 mm and males 9–12 mm in length. *U. stenocephala* females measure 7–12 mm and males 4–5 mm in length (Fig. 2.5).

How do hookworms get into the intestine?

The development of all hookworm species in the environment is similar. Eggs passed in dog or cat faeces contain a group of embryonic cells (morula) from which the larva develops and hatches to become infective after two moults. Infection of the definitive host, the dog or cat, occurs in different ways depending on the species of hookworm and the age of the host animal. For *U. stenocephala*, infection occurs by means of the ingestion of larvae; for *A. caninum*, infection with larvae may occur via the oral, percutaneous or transmammary routes. Hookworms are blood-sucking nematodes that feed on both blood and the intestinal mucosa. Larvae in the environment are the principal source of infection and the main route into puppies for *A. caninum* is transmammary.

Where do hookworms occur?

Hookworms have a worldwide distribution. Their development in the environment is highly temperature and humidity dependent and has been

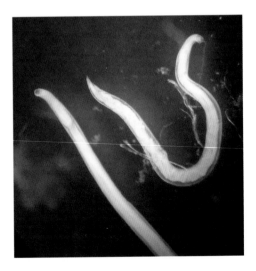

Fig. 2.5. Adult hookworm of dogs, *Uncinaria stenocephala*.

reported to be as short as 6–10 days. *A. caninum* and *A. braziliense* are more prevalent in warmer tropical climates; *U. stenocephala* is well adapted to temperate climates and larvae are even able to survive over winter.

What are the clinical features of hookworm infection in dogs?

Low to medium worm intensities may lead to wasting and reduced growth in puppies. High worm intensities result in diarrhoea containing fresh blood from mucosal lesions and are a cause of death in heavily infected litters. Cutaneous infection with larvae may cause erythema at the penetration sites. The clinical signs that follow are dependent on the migration of the larvae within the body tissue. For example, when larvae reach the brain, ataxia may be seen. *U. stenocephala* and *A. tubaeforme* are less voracious blood feeders than *A. caninum* and *A. braziliense* and as a result worm burdens are better tolerated.

How do you diagnose hookworm infection?

Diagnosis of hookworm infection can be based on faecal flotation/concentration methods. Eggs of *A. caninum* and *U. stenocephala* are soft shelled, containing 4–16-cell morulae in fresh faeces. In general, *A. caninum* eggs (Fig. 2.6a) are shorter and larger in width than those of *U. stenocephala* (Fig. 2.6b). However, although the diagnosis of a hookworm egg is easily done, species determination if required needs some experience based on the appearance of larvae cultured in the laboratory from eggs. In the case of transmammary infection, clinical signs occur in the prepatent period, making diagnosis difficult. *A. caninum* infection should be considered as a differential in any group of puppies suffering from regenerative anaemia

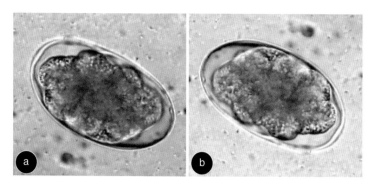

Fig. 2.6. Hookworm eggs. (**a**) Egg of *Ancylostoma caninum*. The egg is oval in shape, thin-shelled, and measures approximately 65 × 40 μm. (**b**) Egg of *Uncinaria stenocephala*. Like eggs of other canine hookworms, *U. stenocephala* eggs are oval or ellipsoidal, thin-shelled, and contain an 8- to 16-cell morula when passed in faeces, but are larger in size (approximately 70–90 μm long × 40–50 μm wide).

and blood loss. Hookworms should also be considered in puppies and kittens as well as adult cats and dogs with mixed worm burdens, diarrhoea and failure to thrive. Polymerase chain reaction (PCR)-based techniques can be used to determine the presence of low worm intensities and permit accurate species identification, but this is performed in research laboratory studies only and is not currently available for general practice. Faecal antigen testing is becoming commercially available, which will provide a sensitive and specific (though comparatively expensive) future (non-routine) alternative to faecal flotation of eggs.

How do you treat and control hookworm infection?

A wide range of anthelmintics is available, such as the MLs and benzimadazoles. Sanitary disposal of dog faeces and prophylactic deworming are also useful in reducing transmission. Numbers of larvae can build up in grassy or damp kennel runs, so using dry concrete flooring in kennels helps to reduce environmental contamination. Treating cats and dogs four times a year is likely to be sufficient to prevent clinical disease in adult pets, though monthly deworming treatments may be desirable to prevent egg production in kennelled situations. Check the websites of Centers for Disease Control and Prevention (CDC) in the USA (www.cdc.gov), CAPC in the USA (www.petsandparasites.org) and ESCCAP in Europe (www.esccap.org) for up-to-date recommendations.

What are the public health implications of hookworms?

Cutaneous larva migrans in humans, also known as 'creeping eruption', is a dermatitis caused by migrating hookworm larvae. Cutaneous larva migrans is a self-limited eruption, as the larvae cannot complete their life cycles in the human body and typically die within 2–8 weeks. However, rare cases lasting up to a year have been reported. Cutaneous larva migrans typically presents with isolated dermatological symptoms. Rare cases associated with Löffler syndrome (the accumulation of eosinophils in the lungs arising from parasitic disease characterized by migratory pulmonary infiltrates and peripheral eosinophilia) have been reported. Two proposed mechanisms for pulmonary involvement include direct invasion of the lungs by the helminths and a systemic immunological process triggered by the helminths, resulting in eosinophilic pulmonary infiltration. The infection is typically acquired in warm climates and tropical areas after coming into direct contact with sand or soil that is contaminated with animal faeces. Therefore, the eruption most commonly occurs as a single or unilateral erythematous, pruritic, serpiginous tract on the feet, hands, or buttocks. The larval tract typically migrates at a rate of 1–2 cm/day, which is in contrast to the serpiginous urticarial rash of larva currens of strongyloidosis (caused by another worm, *Strongyloides* spp.) that can travel up to 10 cm/h.

Whipworm Infection (Trichuriosis)

What are whipworms?

Whipworms are parasitic roundworms, with a very long thin anterior end and a thick tail (approximately 1 cm) giving the worm and overall shape like a whip (Fig. 2.7). The worms live in the small intestines of dogs and other mammals. Whipworms hatch and live in the large intestine throughout their lives and attach themselves to the mucosa, feeding off mucosal epithelium blood and other tissue fluids. Canine whipworms (*Trichuris vulpis*) are found throughout the USA and sporadically in the UK, particularly in kennelled environments, but are most common in warm and humid climates.

How are whipworms spread?

Whipworm eggs are present in the dog waste from infected dogs. Dogs are infected when they consume infective eggs, which occurs most frequently when cleaning their paws or drinking infected water. Different whipworm species have evolved in different animals: those that live in dogs cannot infect people.

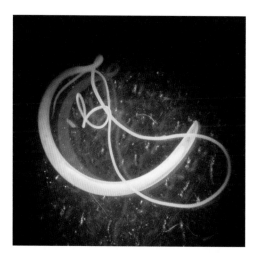

Fig. 2.7. The canine whipworm, *Trichuris vulpis*. Adult worms are characterized by a long thin anterior end that lies in a burrow in the host gut mucosa, and thicker end that extends into the intestinal lumen.

What is the life cycle of whipworms?

The life cycle is direct. Adult males and females live in the colon; eggs are passed in the faeces. The eggs are very resistant to external environmental conditions and can survive for up to 6 years in the environment. Eggs embryonate in the environment in about 3 weeks and an infective L1 larva develops inside the egg. The infective stage is the first-stage larva actually within the egg, which when ingested and digested out of the egg will penetrate the crypts of Lieberkuhn in the colon and become intracellular for several days. Then, larvae develop from L1 to L2 to L3 finally to adults as they move from the base of the crypt to the superficial mucosa. Adult worms maintain their place in the colon by having their anterior end buried in the superficial mucosa.

What are the clinical signs of whipworm infection?

Dogs infected with whipworms generally do not display many signs. The most common visible signs that dogs are clinically infected include bloody stools, weight loss, dehydration and anaemia. While rare, the severe dehydration and anaemia caused by acute whipworm infections may result in the death of the infected animal. Young dogs and puppies are most susceptible to dangerous infections.

What are the pathological findings in dogs with whipworms?

The faeces may contain blood-stained mucus and strips of necrotic mucosa. The nematodes lie with their thin anterior end superficially embedded in the wall of the caecum. The activities of the worms produce little tissue reaction *per se* but enable microorganisms in the gut microflora to become invasive. In high-intensity infections a severe colitis and typhlitis occur, resulting in pseudonecrotic membranes and potentially life-threatening sloughing of colonic mucosa.

How do you diagnose whipworm infections?

Diagnosis of patent whipworm infection is performed by using a faecal flotation test to look for characteristic lemon-shaped eggs. Infections will be missed by flotation tests unless a salt solution of sufficient specific gravity is used; and repeat tests are advised due to intermittent shedding of eggs. Even then, as for many faecal tests, sensitivity may be low. The light-brown oval eggs have a transparent symmetrically opposed plug at each end (Fig. 2.8). At necropsy, the adult worms, which are 2–5 cm long, are easily recognized by their whip-like appearance – the anterior two-thirds are much thinner than the handle-like posterior end.

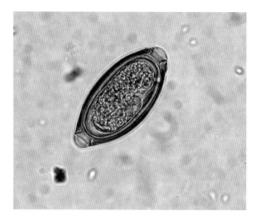

Fig. 2.8. Egg of *Trichuris vulpis*. It has a lemon (or barrel) shape with characteristic plugs at both ends, giving it a tea-tray appearance.

How do you treat and prevent Trichuris *infection?*

Like many parasite eggs in the environment, such as those of *Toxocara* spp., whipworm eggs are extremely tough and difficult to destroy. Indeed, whipworm eggs can live up to 5 years in soil. This means that even if a dog is free of the parasite, reinfection is likely to occur if the immediate environment is contaminated with eggs. The long lifespan of the eggs and subsequent and predictable reinfection means that single whipworm treatments will not control infectious outbreaks. All in-contact dogs should be treated with an effective anthelmintic, such as the benzimadazole, fenbendazole, or the MLs milbemycin oxime or moxidectin, followed by a further dose a month later. Kennelled dogs kept in close proximity may require monthly deworming to keep infection controlled, and kennel runs should be kept dry and grass-free. Faecal contamination should also be kept to a minimum. Routine deworming four times a year with an effective anthelmintic should be sufficient to control clinically significant *T. vulpis* infections in domestic dogs.

Can whipworms of dogs infect humans?

No. Many animals, including humans, have whipworms but they are different species and are host-specific.

Tapeworm Infection

How many tapeworm types infect dogs and cats?

Dogs and cats can be host to parasites belonging to the two major groups of cestodes, namely cyclophyllideans (true cestodes) and pseudophyllideans (pseudo cestodes) (Table 2.1). True cestodes are more commonly encountered.

Table 2.1. Common cestodes in dogs and cats.

Parasite species	Dog or cat	Intermediate host	Infective stage
Cyclophyllidean cestodes:			
Dipylidium caninum	Both	Fleas, lice	Cysticercoid
Taenia species (*see* Table 2.2)	Both	Rabbit and ruminants (definitive host – dogs) Rodents (definitive host – cats)	Cysticercus
Mesocestoides species	Both	Non-fish vertebrates	Tetrathyridium
Echinococcus granulosus *E. multilocularis*	Both	Ruminants (definitive host – dogs). Rodents (definitive host – fox, dogs, coyotes, cats)	Hydatid cyst Alveolar echinococcus
Pseudophyllidean cestodes:			
Spirometra species	Both	Non-fish vertebrates (amphibians, reptiles)	Plerocercoid
Diphyllobothrium latum	Both	Fish	Plerocercoid

How many Taenia *species infect dogs and cats?*

There are several species of genus *Taenia* that can infect dogs and one species that infects cats (Table 2.2). Prepatent period varies according to the species but it generally ranges from 6 to 10 weeks. Depending on species, mature worms can reach up to 5 m in length.

What are the main epidemiological distributions of tapeworms of dogs and cats?

The species of tapeworm found in dogs and cats depends on their geographical location and the amount of free-ranging activity the animals can have. Hence, hunting dogs or cats are at higher risk of infections, while puppies or kittens are less likely to be carrying tapeworms because infection, with the exception of *Dipylidium caninum*, is acquired via eating prey or ruminant offal. *Echinococcus granulosus* is found in limited areas in the UK, including Wales and the Hebridean islands (Fig. 2.9a). All cestodes of dogs and cats have an intermediate host (IH) in which the larval stage develops.

What is the life cycle of tapeworms of dogs and cats?

The common cestodes that infect pets shed egg-laden proglottids (body segments) (Fig. 2.9b) in their faeces. When the appropriate IH ingests these eggs,

Table 2.2. Common *Taenia* species reported in dogs and cats.

Taenia species	Definitive host	Intermediate host	Larval stage and site
T. pisiformis	Dogs and wild canids	Rabbit	*Cysticercus pisiformis* Liver/body cavities
T. hydatigena	Dogs and wild canids	Ruminants (cattle, sheep, deer, elk and moose)	*Cysticercus tenuicollis* Liver/abdominal cavity
T. multiceps	Dogs and wild canids	Sheep and cattle	*Coenurus cerebralis* Central nervous system
T. ovis	Dogs and wild canids	Ruminants (cattle, sheep, deer, elk and moose)	*Cysticercus ovis* Muscles
T. serialis	Dogs and wild canids	Rabbit	*Coenurus serialis* Connective tissues
T. krabbei	Dogs and wild canids	Reindeer	*Cysticercus tarandi* Muscles/abdominal cavity
T. taeniaeformis	Cats	Mice, rats and other small rodents	*Strobilocercus fasciolaris* Liver

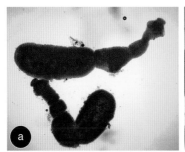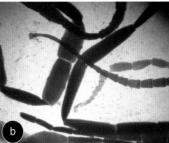

Fig. 2.9. Tapeworms (cestodes). (**a**) The hydatid tapeworm, *Echinococcus granulosus*. (**b**) The flea tapeworm, *Dipylidium caninum*.

larval cysts develop. Dogs and cats are infected when they ingest the IH that contains these larval cysts. These animals may then begin to shed proglottids (in the case of *D. caninum* or *Mesocestoides* spp., as soon as 2–3 weeks after infection). For *Taenia* and *Echinococcus* species, the prepatent period may be as long as 1–2 months. In contrast, adult pseudophyllidean cestodes, such as *Spirometra* spp. or *Diphyllobothrium latum*, discharge individual operculated eggs through a median genital pore in the segment. These eggs hatch upon contact with water and develop in a copepod first IH and a vertebrate second IH before being ingested by a cat or dog definitive host and developing into an adult tapeworm. Dogs and cats may begin to shed pseudophyllidean tapeworm eggs as soon as 10 days after infection. Infections will only occur when dogs and cats ingest larvae in prey species or in undercooked animal tissue in an area where infection is cycling in nature.

What are the clinical features of dogs or cats infected with tapeworms?

Disease in dogs and cats due to infection with adult cyclophyllidean cestodes is rare. Most of tapeworm infections are subclinical. However, heavy infection may occasionally cause disease such as intestinal disturbance, failure to thrive and anaemia. Ulceration and mild inflammation of intestinal mucosa at the site of attachment may be seen on necropsy but the clinical significance of this is often not clear. Also, passage of proglottids may be associated with perianal irritation. Motile segments can be seen on the animal's coat.

How do you diagnose dogs or cats infected with tapeworms?

Diagnosis of *Taenia* and *D. caninum* infection is normally made by finding the proglottids, or chain of proglottids, around the host's anal region or on its fur. Eggs in faeces have a distinctive thick, striated shell but may float poorly in standard faecal flotation solutions, such as sodium chloride or sucrose solutions. When freshly shed, *D. caninum* proglottids have rounded edges like grains of rice, whereas *Taenia* proglottids are more rectangular with sharp corners. Often, *D. caninum* or *Taenia* infection is diagnosed based on a client's observation of proglottids, on or around the pet, that can be motile when fresh or appear like grains of rice when desiccated. *Taenia* tapeworms have one genital opening per proglottid, whereas *D. caninum* has two – one on either side. Further identification of *Taenia* beyond the genus designation can be achieved via morphological characterization of the internal structures, but this is a specialist task. *E. granulosus* eggs cannot be differentiated from *Taenia* eggs (Fig. 2.10a) and faecal flotations carry a poor sensitivity for their detection, making diagnosis difficult. Coproantigen testing carries a high sensitivity for *E. granulosus* and *E. multilocularis* but is not commercially available and is usually reserved for screening or epidemiological studies. *D. caninum* eggs, if observed in faeces, occur in packets contained within a thin-walled membrane, but may be seen as free eggs (Fig. 2.10b,c).

How do you treat dogs or cats infected with tapeworms?

Several treatments are available for the treatment of tapeworm infections in dogs and cats, e.g. praziquantel, epsiprantel or fenbendazole. Praziquantel and epsiprantel are considered the treatments of choice because they are highly effective against *D. caninum*, the most common tapeworm of dogs and cats, as well as *Taenia* spp. and *Echinococcus* spp.

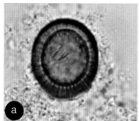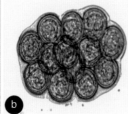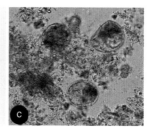

Fig. 2.10. Tapeworm eggs. (a) Typical taeniid's egg, which is morphologically similar between tapeworms of the genus *Taenia* and genus *Echinococcus*. (b) Egg packet of the flea tapeworm *Dipylidium caninum*. (c) Often egg packs will break up and individual eggs will be observed in faeces (each egg is about 40–60 µm in size).

What control measures are advisable for tapeworms of dogs and cats?

Maintenance of *Taenia* and *Echinococcus* depends on pets gaining access to infected prey or ruminant tissues (in the case of rural dogs) or being exposed to fleas (*D. caninum*). Thus, treatment of tapeworms in dogs and cats must be combined with appropriate control measures and husbandry modifications, such as effective flea control and prevention of hunting, for example, to restrict access to the infective larval forms of the cestode. In the absence of these measures, reinfection is likely to occur. Control depends on the tapeworm species. For example, the presence of *D. caninum* necessitates control of fleas and lice. With *Taenia* spp., dogs and cats should not be allowed access to the flesh or viscera of infected intermediate hosts.

Preventing predation and scavenging activity by keeping cats indoors and dogs confined to a leash will limit the opportunity for pets to acquire infection with *Taenia*, *Echinococcus*, *Spirometra* or *D. latum* through ingestion of intermediate hosts. Because scavenging and hunting behaviours can be difficult to prevent totally and because of the difficulties of diagnosing *Echinococcus* infections, which are severe zoonoses, routine monthly deworming of dogs and cats with a broadly cestocidal compound may be indicated, particularly for dogs and cats in areas endemic for *Echinococcus*. *E. multilocularis* is not endemic in the UK but is found in many European countries. Because of its serious zoonotic potential, the praziquantel requirement of the Pet Travel Scheme (PETS) was instigated to treat dogs and cats prior to entry to the UK to keep this zoonotic cestode out of the UK. The 5-day window for praziquantel treatment on the scheme means that there is an opportunity for infection in this time period and dogs entering *E. multilocularis*-free countries should be treated again within 30 days after arrival to ensure that they are free from infection.

Spirocercosis

What is spirocercosis?

Canine spirocercosis is the disease caused by the nematode *Spirocerca lupi*, a spiruroid worm inhabiting granulomatous nodules in the oesophagus of canids and, rarely, felids. The parasite has a worldwide distribution but is most prevalent in warm climates, with high prevalence of infection in South Africa and the Middle East. It is not currently thought to be endemic in the UK, though two individual subclinical infections were recently diagnosed in an untravelled UK cat and dog.

How does S. lupi *reach the oesophagus?*

The adult *S. lupi* is found in a nodular mass in the wall of the host's thoracic oesophagus. The female lays embryonated eggs that are transferred through a tract in the nodule and excreted in the host's faeces. Eggs are ingested by the intermediate host, usually coprophagous beetles, and develop to the infective (L3) stage within 2 months. Carnivores are infected by ingesting a beetle or various paratenic hosts, including birds, hedgehogs, lizards, mice and rabbits. In the carnivore host, the infective larvae penetrate the gastric mucosa and migrate within the walls of the gastric arteries to the thoracic aorta. About 3 months post infection, the larvae leave the aorta and migrate to the oesophagus, where they provoke the development of granulomas as they mature to adults over the next 3 months. The lesions caused by *S. lupi* are mainly due to the migration and persistent presence of larvae and adults in the tissues.

What pathologies are associated with S. lupi?

One of the more interesting pathologies associated with *S. lupi* infection is the induction of oesophageal neoplasms. Oesophageal nodular masses and granulomas and aortic scars and aneurysms are the most frequent lesions. Spondylitis and spondylosis of the caudal thoracic vertebrae are additional typical lesions. Neoplastic transformation of the granulomas to fibrosarcoma or osteosarcoma has been reported in dogs with spirocercosis. As these oesophageal sarcomas enlarge, they may incite the paraneoplastic syndrome known as hypertrophic pulmonary osteoarthropy. In this syndrome, a space-occupying mass in the thorax results in diffuse bony proliferation within the periosteum circumferentially around the diaphyses of bones of the limbs. The exact cause of this new bone formation is obscure but is associated with increased blood flow to the limbs early in the disease course. Less frequently, lesions may occur due to the aberrant migration of the worms. *S. lupi* worms and nodules have been reported in thoracic organs, the gastrointestinal tract, the urinary system and subcutaneous tissues. Aortic nodules associated with larvae may become aneurysms, which occasionally rupture leading to haemorrhage and death.

Do dogs with spirocercosis exhibit clinical signs?

The clinical signs depend on the location and severity of the lesions. Oesophageal lesions are associated with persistent vomiting and/or regurgitation followed by weakness and emaciation. Sudden death may be caused by rupture of an aortic nodule. Spinal pain may be associated with bony proliferation.

How do you diagnose dogs with spirocercosis?

A definite diagnosis of spirocercosis is made by detection of characteristic small (11–15 × 30–38 μm) larvated eggs by faecal flotation. Thoracic radiographs of affected dogs show oesophageal granulomas as areas of increased density in the caudodorsal mediastinum and contrast oesophograms may outline granulomas. Oesophagoscopy and gastroscopy allow direct visualization of the nodules, which appear as broad-based protuberances with a distinct nipple-like orifice.

How do you manage a dog with spirocercosis?

Several anthelmintics have been suggested for the treatment of canine spirocercosis, including diethylcarbamazine, disophenol, levamizole, albendazole, ivermectin and doramectin. Moxidectin is now licensed in Europe for treatment of *S. lupi* infection as a spot-on solution in dogs (in combination with imidacloprid) with excellent management of oesophageal lesions that have not progressed to malignancy. Surgical excision of oesophageal granulomas and sarcomas is often not possible, due to extensive or multiple lesions. Contact with intermediate hosts should ideally be avoided but this is difficult to achieve in pets with access to outdoor environments, particularly given the wide range of paratenic hosts that may be infected.

Stomach Worm *Ollulanus tricuspis* Infection

What sort of worm is *Ollulanus tricuspis*?

O. tricuspis is a small nematode of the stomach of cats and other mammals. It is notable by its size (≤ 1 cm), spiral coil of the head and the presence of a copulatory bursa in males and three to four short tooth-like structures (cusps) on the tail of female (Fig. 2.11). *O. tricuspis* has a worldwide distribution but appears to be rare, mainly occurring in Europe, the Americas, Australia and the Middle East.

How do adult *O. tricuspis* get into the stomach?

The parasite has a highly unusual and direct life cycle. The females are viviparous, i.e. eggs hatch and larval development to infective L3 occurs inside the uterus of the female. The whole cycle can be completed endogenously in the same cat. Infective L3s are released into the lumen of the stomach and develop into adults on the gastric mucosa in around 4–5 weeks. The L3s

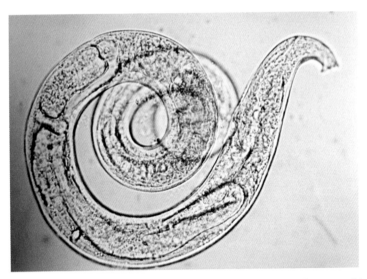

Fig. 2.11. Female *Ollulanus tricuspis* worm. Adult measures 0.8–1 mm long; its tail has five cusps. These worms live in the stomach and may burrow into the gastric mucosa.

may be transmitted to another cat through contact with vomit from an infected cat. Adult worms normally live under a layer of mucus in the stomach wall but they may burrow into the gastric mucosa, leading to gastritis. Hypertrophic to fibrosing gastritis has been reported. Sometimes, no macroscopic lesions can be seen in the stomachs of infected cats.

Are there clinical signs associated with O. tricuspis infection?

O. tricuspis causes increased mucus production, anorexia, intermittent vomiting, emaciation and haematemesis. Severe chronic gastritis and occasional death have been reported in heavily infected cats and other felids.

How do you diagnose O. tricuspis infection?

Diagnosis is made by identification of tiny larvae and adult worms in the vomit or stomach contents, or in scrapings collected by gastric lavage. The Baermann apparatus can be used to concentrate worms in vomitus.

How do you treat an O. tricuspis infection?

Fenbendazole, levamisole or ivermectin can be effective. Control includes good sanitation and prevention of contact with the vomit of infected cats.

What are the public health implications of O. tricuspis?

There is no evidence that this worm is zoonotic.

Giardiosis

What is giardiosis?

Giardiosis is an intestinal protozoal disease caused by *Giardia duodenalis* (synonyms *G. lamblia* and *G. intestinalis*) infection. The life cycle of *G. duodenalis* is similar in dogs, cats and humans. *Giardia* parasites have two life cycle forms, cysts and trophozoites, which are shed in the faeces of infected animals or humans. Infection occurs either after the ingestion of cysts through the faecal–oral route or after the ingestion of contaminated food or water.

What tests are available for diagnosis of giardiosis?

Diagnosis is by detection of *Giardia* cysts (Fig. 2.12) and occasionally trophozoites in the faeces of affected animals. However, giardiosis is often difficult to diagnose, because many of the signs are non-specific and because of the low sensitivity of microscopic methods (e.g. examination of faecal smears). This is due to the small size and low numbers of cysts present in the faeces and the intermittent shedding of these cysts. Sensitivity is improved if samples are collected over a 3-day period. A *Giardia* faecal enzyme-linked immunosorbent assay (ELISA) test kit is available in some countries, and the SNAP® *Giardia* Test kit (IDEXX Laboratories) is a relatively new rapid enzyme immunoassay – a point-of-use test – for the detection of *Giardia* antigen in canine and feline faeces. Positive results indicate the presence of antigen of *Giardia* trophozoites or cysts in the intestine. Care must be taken interpreting a positive result, as antigen may still be shed after infection has been eliminated.

Is giardiosis in dogs and cats considered zoonotic?

Current opinion suggests that the genotypic subgroup predominantly affecting humans is different from two other distinct subgroups predominantly affecting cats and dogs. While the human *Giardia* genotype can readily

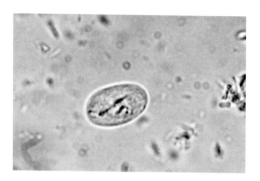

Fig. 2.12. Cyst of the intestinal protozoan *Giardia duodenalis*. Approximately 12 microns.

infect other mammals, it is thought that infection of people with cat and dog *Giardia* genotypes is more difficult and this is borne out by the high prevalence of *Giardia* infection in cats and dogs (as high as 50% in some studies) in the UK but the relatively low prevalence of *Giardia* in people in the UK. This allows us to draw the following practical conclusions about transmission of *Giardia* between pets and people.

1. Pets of any species that are infected with *Giardia* do not pose a high zoonotic risk as long as their owners have not already been infected. However, the zoonotic risk they do pose has not been quantified and so advising good hygiene to owners and treatment of their pets to eliminate the parasite is still very important in minimizing any zoonotic risk that may be present.

2. Human giardiosis may be cycled through pets, allowing transmission to other people. An example would be if a person contracted *Giardia* infection abroad and then visited friends who had pets. Although the infected person may exercise strict hygiene around food and communal items, it would be very easy for pets in the household to become infected and then pass on the disease to other people. Under these circumstances rapid identification of infected people and pets is vital so that rapid chemotherapeutic elimination of the parasite can be achieved. This is in addition to strict hygiene.

3. In the same manner, people infected with *Giardia* who work with domestic animals pose a high risk of infecting animals that may then remain a reservoir of infection for people. This reservoir of infection may remain undetected in the long term if the carrier animals remain subclinical. As a result, there is a strong case for people working in the veterinary profession who have been infected with the parasite being isolated from pets at work until the infection has been cleared. Infected people also have the potential to infect wild animals through water or soil contamination during camping and other outdoor pursuits. These animals can then infect large numbers of people through contamination of domestic water supplies. Infected people or owners of infected pets seeking advice should be made aware of the risk of widespread infection through faecal water contamination. Therefore, diagnosis and awareness of giardiosis in animals is important, not only to treat clinical cases, but also to prevent transmission to other animals and humans by practising good hand hygiene and, where practical, elimination of infection.

How is giardiosis treated?

Fenbendazole at 50 mg/kg for 5 days is effective in improving clinical signs and may eliminate infection. Supportive treatment may also be required for the diarrhoea. Some infections are persistent despite prolonged courses of treatment. Where elimination of the parasite is desirable to limit further spread and any zoonotic risk, there is some evidence to suggest that combining fenbendazole treatment with metronidazole is more effective at eliminating shedding than fenbendazole alone.

Is resistance developing in Giardia to fenbendazole? Should confirmed infection always be treated?

Cases of suspected resistance to fenbendazole have been reported in North America and there has been subsequent debate about whether diagnosed *Giardia* infections should be treated, given that many are subclinical and that in many cases zoonotic risk is limited. If *Giardia* infection is diagnosed with concurrent clinical signs, then treatment should be initiated for 5 days. If signs resolve and infection is still present, then ongoing treatment to eliminate infection and whether it is warranted should be discussed with the owner.

How do you protect dogs against giardiosis?

Prevention of *Giardia* infection in dogs depends upon the quick removal of faecal material, preventing dogs from consuming contaminated surface water or faeces, and the disinfection and cleaning of kennels. The disinfection of kennels can be accomplished with 1% sodium hypochlorite (20% commercial bleach), 2% glutaraldehyde or quaternary ammonium compounds. Cysts are relatively resistant to chlorination and levels of chlorine in drinking water are inadequate to inactivate cysts. However, *Giardia* cysts are susceptible to desiccation, and cleaning and thorough drying will kill them.

Tritrichomonosis

What is feline intestinal tritrichomonosis?

Feline intestinal tritrichomonosis is caused by the protozoan *Tritrichomonas foetus*, which has recently attracted attention as a cause of chronic large-bowel diarrhoea and poor body condition. The perineum and hind limbs are stained with yellow faecal material. Motile flagellated trophozoites of trichomonads, featuring a pear-shaped body with an undulating membrane and three free anterior flagella, are sometimes visible on direct microscopic examination of a rectal faecal swab.

How do cats become infected with this parasite and what are the risk factors for infection?

Transmission from cat to cat is by the faecal–oral route. The disease is mainly seen in densely housed young cats (i.e. where faecal–oral transmission may readily occur), cats living in multi-cat households (catteries or shelters) and young pedigree cats.

What other laboratory tests are required to confirm this infection?

Tests include microscopic examination of wet mounts of freshly voided faeces (Fig. 2.13), faecal culture in selective media (e.g. InPouch™, TF-Feline medium), colonic/ileal biopsy and immune-histochemistry or faecal PCR on pooled faeces over 3 days. Testing for *T. foetus* should form part of the routine work-up of chronic diarrhoea in cats, particularly in young purebred cats and cats with large-bowel diarrhoea.

How do you treat this infection?

Metronidazole and fenbendazole only cause temporary remission of clinical signs and should be avoided. Some clinical cases are self-limiting but, if required, tritrichomonosis can be successfully treated with ronidazole (30–50 mg/kg once or twice a day for 14 days); the use of this drug is off-label and close monitoring is mandatory, because cats treated with high doses may exhibit neurological signs. Also, introduction of a high-fibre diet, reduction of environmental stress, optimizing litter tray hygiene and treating or isolating in-contact cats will help to limit clinical signs and control spread of infection.

Can this parasite infect people?

Yes, though human cases are extremely rare. People in contact with infected cats are advised to take basic hygiene precautions to avoid ingesting the

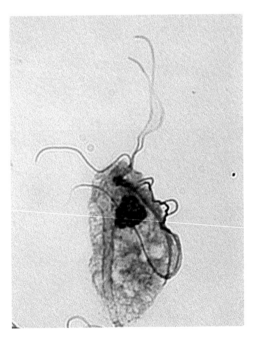

Fig. 2.13. Feline intestinal protozoan *Tritrichomonas foetus*. It measures 10 to 26 μm.

parasite. Cat scratches or bites should always be washed immediately with soap and water. Anyone with a weakened immune system should not handle cat faeces or litter boxes.

Acanthocephalan Infection

What are acanthocephalans?

Acanthocephalans are found in many species of fish, amphibians, birds and mammals. Several morphological characteristics serve to separate acanthocephalans from other parasitic worms but probably the most notable is the presence of an anterior protrusible proboscis that is usually covered with small hooks (Fig. 2.14). It is this characteristic that gives the acanthocephalans their common name, the 'thorny-headed worms'. The life cycles of all acanthocephalans appear to follow the same basic pattern. The adult acanthocephalans occur in the intestine of the definitive host. The sexes are separate, i.e. they are dioecious, and the females produce eggs that are passed in the host's faeces. The eggs are ingested by an intermediate host, an arthropod, in which the parasite goes through several developmental or juvenile stages. The definitive host is infected with the parasite when it eats an intermediate host containing the parasite.

The acanthocephalan *Oncicola canis* can be found in the small intestine of dogs and cats. It is white and approximately 8–15 mm long, and the thorny head is embedded in the mucosa. *Macracanthorhynchus ingens*, another acanthocephalan, is a parasite of raccoons but may occasionally infect dogs and perforate the gut, causing peritonitis. The adult males are 10 cm long and the females are up to 35 cm long. It has unique spindle-shaped eggs (91 μm length × 54 μm width).

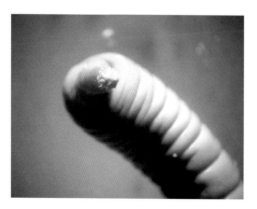

Fig. 2.14. Acanthocephalan worm, also called 'thorny-headed worm' due to the presence of protrusible proboscis armed with hooks, the main morphological feature that separates acanthocephalans from other parasitic worms.

Self-Assessment Questions

1. **Which of the following routes of *Toxocara* spp. transmission is not significant in cats?**

    (a) Transplacental

    (b) Transmammary

    (c) Ingestion of embryonated eggs

    (d) Ingestion of paratenic hosts

2. **What is the minimum recommended worming frequency for *Toxocara canis*?**

    (a) Once a year

    (b) Every 6 months

    (c) Every 4 months

    (d) Every 3 months

3. **Cutaneous larval migrans is caused predominantly by which type of worm?**

    (a) Hookworm

    (b) *Toxocara* spp.

    (c) Tapeworm

    (d) Whipworm

4. ***Ollulanus tricuspis* infects which part of the digestive tract?**

    (a) Oesophagus

    (b) Stomach

    (c) Small intestine

    (d) Colon

5. ***Spirocerca lupi* infects which part of the digestive tract?**

    (a) Oesophagus

    (b) Stomach

    (c) Small intestine

    (d) Colon

3 Parasites of the Respiratory System

Angiostrongylosis (*Angiostrongylus vasorum*)

What is canine angiostrongylosis?

This parasitic worm infects dogs and the infective L3 larvae are carried by slugs and snails. Referring to *Angiostrongylus vasorum* as a lungworm is something of a misnomer. Although the larval and egg stages of the parasite do affect the lungs and coughing associated with bronchitis is the most common presenting sign, the adult worms actually live in the heart and pulmonary artery. *A. vasorum* is also known as the French heartworm but the term heartworm should really be for *Dirofilaria immitis*, covered in the next chapter.

Infections in dogs may be subclinical or lead to clinical pathology and signs (angiostrongylosis) including bronchitis, clotting defects, neurological deficits associated with blood clots and aberrant larval migration and heart disease. Secondary coagulopathies (disseminated intravascular coagulation, immune-mediated thrombocytopenia) can result in subcutaneous haematomas or occasionally in fatal cerebral, spinal or abdominal haemorrhage. Ascites, syncope, vomiting and signs of central nervous system disease may also occur. On rare occasions sudden death after an acute onset of clinical disease can occur, usually in younger dogs.

In the UK, this disease was largely confined to dogs living in the south of the country in the 1990s (especially the south-east and south-west of England and south Wales) but in the past 10 years the disease has become much more common and has been seen in dogs as far north as Scotland. The possibility of exposure and subsequent infection should therefore now be considered in all UK dogs. *A. vasorum* is also increasing its range within many other European countries as well as parts of Africa and South America, and in a single focus in North America in Canada (Newfoundland). The natural definitive hosts are various species of fox that act as reservoirs of infection. Given the ease and frequency of travel within North America coupled with the presence of a large red fox population and the abundance of gastropod intermediate hosts, it seems highly likely that the endemic range of *A. vasorum* will spread from Newfoundland to other parts of North America, as well as consolidating and increasing its range in the UK and Europe as a whole.

How are domestic dogs infected?

The adult worms spend most of their lives in the blood vessels close to the heart. However, when eggs are laid, they move through the lung parenchyma and hatch out as first-stage (L1) larvae. The larvae travel through the lungs and the dog then coughs them up and swallows them. These L1 larvae pass into the faeces and, when eaten by slugs and snails, moult twice to the infective L3 stage. Slugs are the most important intermediate hosts since they are coprophagic detritivores, highly attracted to faecal matter. There is some debate concerning possible additional routes of infection for pet dogs, besides actually eating an infected mollusc. For example, slugs and snails often crawl into dogs' food bowls or on to toys if these are left outside, and if ingested by the dog, the lungworms continue their life cycle. Dogs also eat these garden pests when drinking from outdoor water sources and eating grass. Whatever the route, once ingested, infective larvae move to the gut where they penetrate the gut wall and enter the bloodstream and lymphatic system and eventually reach the right side of the heart, where they become adult worms. Here, the adult releases eggs that hatch in the blood and then make their way to the lungs, rupturing the lung wall, entering the alveoli (the tiny air pockets in the lungs) and working their way up through the lungs (Fig. 3.1) until they reach the top. This makes the dog cough, bringing up the lungworms. The dog swallows them and passes them through the digestive tract to exit the body in faeces. Frogs may also act as intermediate hosts. The prepatent period varies from 28 to 108 days.

How do you know if a dog is infected?

Many infected dogs show no signs of illness. Dogs that are unwell show a wide range of clinical signs including breathing problems, coughing, bleeding excessively from cuts or bleeding internally with no signs of trauma, but with anaemia and loss of condition. Other animals may show neurological changes, including seizures. *A. vasorum* should be considered as a differential if dogs present with any of these signs.

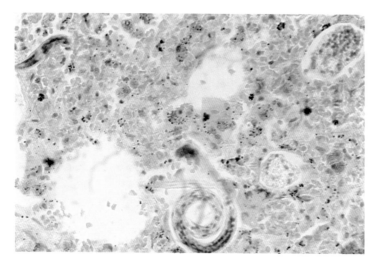

Fig. 3.1. Larvae of the canine lungworm, *Angiostrongylus vasorum*, in lung tissue of a dog.

What is the differential diagnosis for clinical signs associated with A. vasorum *infection?*

Options include heartworm disease (*Dirofilaria immitis*), A. *vasorum* infection, right-sided heart failure and right atrial haemangiosarcoma for cardiac signs and changes, and kennel cough and allergic bronchitis for bronchitic signs. Toxin exposure, genetic predilection and previous history should all be considered for neurological and clotting defect presentations. It is also important to remember that other lungworms besides A . *vasorum* may infect dogs, though they are rarer, and precise identification is needed since associated risk factors, advice provided and the management of lungworm infection is species specific.

How is a diagnosis of A. vasorum *accomplished?*

Detection of A. *vasorum* infection in dogs can be accomplished based on history, clinical signs and laboratory investigation. The latter includes: (i) detection and morphological identification of L1 in faecal samples following concentration using the Baermann technique (the traditional gold-standard method); (ii) cytological examination of samples collected from tracheal wash or bronchoalveolar lavage; (iii) blood profile; (iv) serological assays; and (v) PCR. Definitive diagnosis is by the detection of L1 larvae in faeces or bronchial mucus. Larvae are 310–399 µm in length and the tail terminates in a sinus wave-shaped kink with a prominent dorsal spine (Fig. 3.2). The method of choice for faecal detection of L1 larvae is the Baermann technique.

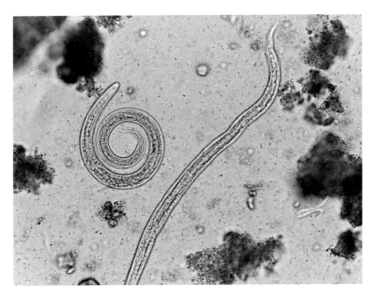

Fig. 3.2. *Angiostrongylus vasorum* larvae recovered from faeces using Baermann method.

A sandwich ELISA for detecting circulating antigens of *A. vasorum* has recently been developed and is now commercially available, with a reported test specificity of 100% and sensitivity of 92%. The presence of radiographic changes (interstitial pattern), reduced serum levels of fructosamine, or calcaemia may also aid in diagnosis. A lateral thoracic radiograph might show multifocal bronchial and peribronchial interstitial and alveolar patterns associated with moderately dilated pulmonary arteries. Radiographic changes seen in *D. immitis* heartworm disease (right-sided cardiomegaly, enlarged main pulmonary artery, dilated and tortuous lobar pulmonary arteries, blunting of pulmonary arteries, enlarged caudal vena cava) are not typically present in *A. vasorum* infection. Also, *D. immitis* that are obvious in the right ventricle (RV) and right atrium (RA) as a mass of short parallel lines on echocardiography are not seen in *A. vasorum* infection. There is no dilation of the RV. An abnormal cardiac silhouette may indicate a mass.

What is the treatment for A. vasorum *infection?*

A number of drugs can be used to eliminate the worms but infected dogs should be monitored carefully when receiving treatment, as the sudden killing of the worms could result in a severe allergic reaction. If the dog has severe signs (particularly affecting the brain or signs of heart failure) the veterinary surgeon will want to keep the dog in the hospital for specialized care. Fenbendazole, milbemycin oxime and moxidectin are all used to treat angiostrongylosis in dogs, with high efficacy. Irrespective of the choice of anthelmintic, post-treatment complications that may involve severe dyspnoea or ascites can occur.

Administration of bronchodilators and diuretics is indicated in these cases. Fenbendazole (20–25 mg/kg, oral, once a day for 20–21 days, or 50 mg/kg, oral, once a day for 5–21 days) has been widely used in naturally infected dogs. Fenbendazole is not licensed in the UK to treat *A. vasorum* but is still widely used, as there are anecdotal reports that daily use of fenbendazole reduces the risk of post-treatment anaphylaxis through 'slow kill' of parasitic stages. There is, however, no peer review evidence to support this. Milbemycin oxime (0.5 mg/kg, oral) given once a week for 4 weeks orally is efficacious and a licensed treatment protocol for *A. vasorum* infection. Similarly, a single topical application of moxidectin (2.5 mg/kg) is licensed to treat *A. vasorum*, with a reported efficacy of 85%. A second treatment 4 weeks later is then sufficient to clear patent infection if this is not achieved by the first treatment. Supportive treatment with antibiotics to treat secondary infection is indicated if supported by cultures. Bronchodilators and corticosteroids are commonly given as symptomatic treatment for clinical signs. Blood transfusion or plasma may also be required to correct blood loss and supply clotting factors. Oxygen supplementation is useful in cases of respiratory compromise. Most dogs go on to make a full recovery with appropriate treatment. However, infection can prove fatal for some dogs despite intensive treatment.

How can A. vasorum *infection be prevented?*

Dogs are infected by ingestion of or contact with slugs or snails, so reducing a dog's exposure to molluscs will reduce the risk of infection. This can be difficult to achieve for dogs with access to outdoor environments; and use of molluscicides can result in increased shedding of infective stages into the environment and dead slugs and snails being consumed. Preventive anthelmintics are therefore the principal strategy for preventing infection, given in the form of monthly oral milbemycin oxime or a monthly moxidectin spot-on treatment at the back of the neck. In the UK the red fox is the most important reservoir of infection and avoiding fox-inhabited areas is desirable but largely impractical.

What are the public health implications of A. vasorum?

There have been no reported cases of *A. vasorum* in humans. Humans can be infected with other *Angiostrongylus* spp., e.g. *A. cantonensis*, in various parts of the world, notably south-east Asia.

Crenosomosis

What is Crenosoma vulpis?

Crenosoma vulpis, the fox lungworm, occurs in the trachea, bronchi and bronchioles of wild and domestic canids in the temperate regions of North America and Europe. Adult worms are 5–10 mm in length and the anterior end is marked by a characteristic series of 18–26 ring-like cuticular folds. The parasite has recently been recognized as an important cause of chronic respiratory disease in dogs in parts of Canada and Europe. In North America, the geographical distribution of *C. vulpis* seems to be mainly in the north-eastern portion of the continent, including parts of the USA and Canada. The North American natural definitive hosts are species of wild canids, including foxes and coyotes. Apart from the Atlantic Canadian provinces, infection in dogs seems to be infrequent in North America. Crenosomosis has been found to be a frequent cause of chronic respiratory disease in dogs, occurring in 21% of dogs showing signs of chronic cough. Canids acquire infection by the ingestion of terrestrial snail and slug gastropod intermediate hosts. The prepatent period is 19–21 days and the infection induces chronic bronchitis–bronchiolitis, which results in clinical signs consisting primarily of chronic cough sometimes accompanied by gagging.

How is crenosomosis diagnosed?

Definitive diagnosis is by detection of first-stage larvae in faeces or transtracheal wash samples. Larvae (Fig. 3.3) are best detected in faeces by Baermann examination or by using the FLOTAC device (recently developed in Italy and available in Europe) but the former seems to be the most sensitive method for diagnosis. As with other metastrongylids, faecal larval

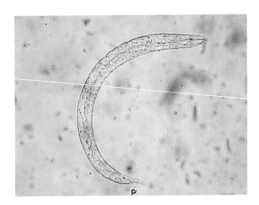

Fig. 3.3. Larva of the fox lungworm, *Crenosoma vulpis*.

shedding may be intermittent and therefore examination of multiple faecal samples (three collected over 7 days) will increase detection sensitivity. Larvae are 264–340 × 16–22 μm in size. The larval tail is pointed and lacks a kink or dorsal spine seen in *A. vasorum.*

How do you treat C. vulpis *infection?*

Febantel (14 mg/kg, oral, once a day for 7 days) and fenbendazole (25–50 mg/kg, oral, once a day for 3–14 days) have been used successfully to treat *C. vulpis* but are not licensed for this use in the UK. Oral milbemycin oxime and moxidectin spot-on treatments have been shown to have efficacy and are licensed for UK use. All these treatments have been used to treat dogs naturally infected with *C. vulpis*, with a clinical cure occurring within 7–10 days of treatment. A treatment efficacy of 98–99% was reported for milbemycin oxime (0.5 mg/kg, oral) used in the treatment of dogs experimentally infected with *C. vulpis*. Crenosomosis may be misdiagnosed as allergic respiratory disease and dogs will show a positive clinical response due to the symptomatic relief of corticosteroid therapy.

Canine Verminous Nodular Bronchitis (*Oslerus osleri*)

What is Oslerus osleri?

O. osleri is a parasite found in the trachea and bronchi of dogs, coyotes and wolves and has a worldwide distribution. In North America and Europe, infection is fairly common and widespread in wild canids, particularly coyotes. However, wild canids do not seem to serve as an infection reservoir for dogs; dogs exposed to infective larvae derived from coyotes failed to develop *O. osleri* infections. Infection in dogs is infrequent but isolated cases have been reported throughout the UK, USA and Canada. Adult worms are 6.5–13.5 mm long and reside coiled inside wart-like nodules that are attached to the mucosal epithelium in the lumen of the trachea and bronchi. The nodules are clustered at the bifurcation of the trachea. Individual nodules range in size from 1 mm to 20 mm and can become confluent when present in large numbers.

How does O. osleri *survive?*

Unusually for a metastrongyloid parasite, the life cycle for *O. oslerus* is direct and the first-stage larva is the infective stage. Adult females lay thin-shelled larvated eggs (80 × 50 μm) that hatch, and the first-stage larvae migrate up the bronchial system to pass either in saliva or in the faeces. Larvae recovered from the faeces tend to be sluggish and are often found to be dead and degenerating. Transmission in wild canids occurs mainly by exposure of weanling puppies by the dam through regurgitative feeding. Transmission in dogs is thought to be mainly through saliva from the dam cleaning her puppies through licking. Exposure can also be through ingestion of larvae from faecal contamination but this is of lesser importance, except in kennel environments where numbers of larvae can build up, leading to clinical outbreaks. Immature worms arrive in the trachea about 70 days after exposure and nodules are visible soon after. The prepatent period is about 92–126 days.

How do you diagnose O. osleri *infection?*

Diagnosis of infection tends to occur in young dogs, 6 months to 2 years old, which is consistent with exposure at an early age. Clinical signs consist of chronic cough, which may be worse with exercise, and in some cases wheezing and dyspnoea occur. Weight loss, emaciation and collapse may be observed in the most severely affected dogs. Pneumothorax was reported in one case of *O. osleri* infection. Infections may be subclinical in some dogs. Definitive diagnosis is by visualization of the nodules at the bifurcation of the trachea with bronchoscopy followed by recovery of first-stage larvae in bronchial mucus or, less commonly, in faeces. Larvae recovered from bronchial mucus are 233–267 μm in length and the tail ends in a distinctive sinus wave-shaped kink (Fig. 3.4), but they lack the distinct dorsal appendage seen in *A. vasorum*. Transtracheal wash samples or bronchial mucus collected during bronchoscopy are superior to faecal detection methods for larval recovery. Zinc sulphate (ZnSO$_4$) centrifugal faecal flotation has a greater sensitivity than Baermann examination; however, false-negative results are a problem with both methods and repeat sequential analysis might be advisable.

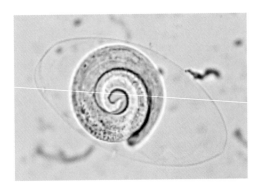

Fig. 3.4. *Filaroides osleri* (formerly *Oslerus osleri*) larva. It has a tail with a short S-shaped appendage. *Filaroides* are unique among nematodes because their first-stage larvae are immediately infective for the dog.

How do you treat O. osleri?

Fenbendazole and ivermectin have been used in naturally infected dogs, with variable results. Fenbendazole is licensed for the treatment of O. *osleri* and treatment at 50 mg/kg, oral, once a day for 7–14 days was reported to be effective in the treatment of 20 dogs with clinical O. *osleri* infections. One severely affected dog required two 14-day courses of the fenbendazole treatment. Ivermectin (0.4 mg/kg, subcutaneous, repeated every 3 weeks for four treatments) was reported to be effective in the treatment of four dogs, resulting in a clinical cure and resolution of tracheobronchial nodules.

Canine Verminous Pneumonia (*Filaroides* spp.)

What are Filaroides?

There are two closely related species, *Filaroides hirthi* and *Filaroides milksi*, occurring in the lung parenchyma of dogs. *F. milksi* (= *Andersonstrongylus milksi*) was first reported as an incidental finding from the necropsy of a 10-year-old Boston terrier. Adult worms (3.4–10.9 mm in length) were found in bronchioles and coiled in nests in the lung parenchyma. *F. hirthi* was first reported, also as an incidental finding at necropsy, in the bronchioles and lung parenchyma of purpose-bred research beagles. Adult worms are 2.3–13 mm in length. The two species are differentiated from each other based on subtle differences in adult worm size and male spicule morphology and length. These parasites are rarely seen in the UK and Europe.

The validity of *F. milksi* and *F. hirthi* as two separate species has been questioned, resulting in some debate. Prevalence of *F. hirthi* infection as high as 78% in individual research dog colonies has been reported but diagnosis in client-owned dogs in the USA is rare, though cases are reported from Alabama, Georgia, New York, Pennsylvania, Texas and Washington. There are fewer reports of *F. milksi* infection. Diagnosis in dogs based on histopathology has been reported in Australia, Canada and the USA; however, differentiation between *F. hirthi* and *F. milksi* is not possible based on histopathology and these may have been *F. hirthi*. In addition to the original species description, there is only one other report of a diagnosis in a dog based on identification of adult male worms. Reports of *F. milksi* infection in the skunk and in a dog from Belgium have been disputed.

How do Filaroides live?

The life cycle is unknown for *F. milksi*. Transmission of *F. hirthi* occurs by ingestion of infective L1 larvae, usually through coprophagia of fresh faecal material. In research beagle colonies this is thought to occur in puppies by 4–5 weeks of age through exposure to faeces from infected dams.

The prepatent period is 35 days. Infections appear to be long lived and this is probably due to re-exposure to infective first-stage larvae through autoinfection. Most infections appear to be subclinical. Most reports involve young (< 3 years) small toy breeds, such as Chihuahua, West Highland Terrier, Toy Poodle and Yorkshire Terrier. Fatal infections have also occurred in dogs up to 10 years old and in such breeds as the King Charles Spaniel and Dalmatian. Clinically affected dogs show signs of dyspnoea, cough and cyanosis and may be depressed.

How do you diagnose Filaroides?

Diagnosis is by detection of first-stage larvae in bronchial mucus or faeces. The larvae of *F. hirthi* and *F. milksi* cannot be differentiated from each other or from those of *O. osleri*. Larvae are 240–290 μm in length and have a kinked tail (Fig. 3.5). Also, in common with *O. osleri*, detection sensitivity of *Filaroides* larvae by Baermann examination is poor. Larvae are best detected by examination of bronchial mucus. Faecal detection can be achieved by flotation in $ZnSO_4$ but larvae are quickly distorted. Additional diagnostics might include radiographs, showing interstitial linear and focal nodular pulmonary infiltrates.

How do you treat Filaroides?

Albendazole, fenbendazole and ivermectin have been used to treat dogs infected with *F. hirthi*. Control in research dog colonies by treating breeding animals using albendazole (25 mg/kg, oral, twice a day for 5 days; repeated in 2–4 weeks) and ivermectin (1 mg/kg, subcutaneous, repeated in 1 week) has been reported. Fenbendazole (50 mg/kg, oral, once a day for 14–21 days

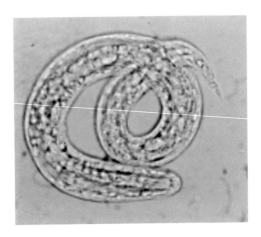

Fig. 3.5. *Filaroides hirthi* larva.

or 100 mg/kg, oral, once a day for 7 days) appeared to be an effective treatment in three dogs. Corticosteroids were used in one of the dogs as an adjunct therapy due to severe post-treatment dyspnoea that was attributed to an inflammatory response to dead worms. Ivermectin (0.034 mg/kg, oral, single dose) followed by fenbendazole (50 mg/kg, oral, once a day for 14 days) appeared to be an effective treatment in one dog.

Eucoleosis

What is Eucoleus aerophilus?

Eucoleus aerophilus (= *Capillaria aerophila*) occurs in the trachea, bronchi and bronchioles, infects dogs, cats and various wild carnivores and has a worldwide distribution. At one time, *E. aerophilus* was also thought to occur sometimes in the nasal passages and sinuses of dogs and wild canids but it is now recognized that this was a second species, *Eucoleus boehmi*. Interpretation of study results from some of the older literature is complicated by the uncertainty about which of the two species the researchers may have been dealing with. *E. aerophilus* worms are long and thin, measuring 16–40 × 0.06–0.18 mm. Reports of prevalence in North America have ranged from 0% to 5% in dogs and 0.2% to 9% in cats. For the UK, this parasite is rarely seen in dogs, but up to 70% of foxes are infected in some regions, according to recent surveys.

The life cycle may be direct or earthworms can serve as a paratenic/intermediate host. Eggs are long-lived in the environment and the prepatent period has been reported as 40 days. Infection in dogs and cats is usually well tolerated; however, chronic cough can develop that may also lead to loss of weight and body condition, and rarely ends in death. Definitive diagnosis is by detection of eggs on faecal flotation. The eggs have bipolar plugs, asymmetrically opposed, and measure 58–79 × 29–40 μm in size (Fig. 3.6). These eggs, the shell wall surface of which is unusual in having a netlike pattern, may also be detected in bronchoalveolar lavage samples. Other diagnostic tests, suggestive of but non-specific for *E. aerophilus* infection, include radiographs indicating a diffuse interstitial lung pattern and transtracheal wash cytology showing an eosinophilic inflammatory response.

What is E. boehmi?

E. boehmi occurs in the nasal passages and sinuses of wild and domestic canids in Europe, North America and South America. The worms are long and thin (22–43 mm × 0.08–0.15 mm) and are found embedded in the epithelial lining of the nasal turbinates, frontal sinuses and paranasal sinuses. The life cycle and routes of transmission are unknown. Earthworms may serve

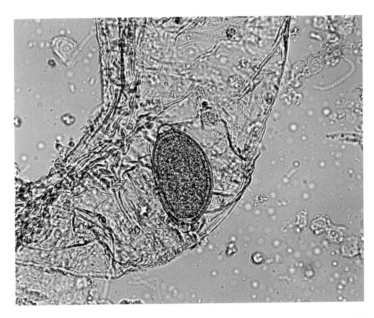

Fig. 3.6. Egg of *Capillaria aerophila* with its characteristic bipolar plugs (asymmetrical) and rough surface ('netted' in appearance).

as intermediate hosts but further study is required to confirm this. Clinically affected dogs show signs of sneezing and mucopurulent nasal discharge that may contain blood. Faecal flotation survey results usually do not differentiate between capillarid species, therefore little is known on prevalence and distribution of *E. boehmi* infection in canids in North America. Only 0.4% of 6458 canine faecal samples tested in a national faecal flotation survey in the USA were positive for capillarid eggs, most of which were *E. boehmi*. Positive samples were recorded from each of the regions sampled. A faecal flotation survey of greyhounds in Kansas detected eggs of *E. boehmi* in 2% (4 of 230) of the samples.

Diagnosis is based on detection of eggs in faeces by faecal flotation. Egg shedding may be cyclical, therefore multiple faecal examinations may be needed to detect infection. Eggs may also be detected by microscopic examination of nasal discharge. The eggs are bipolar plugged, contain a multi-celled embryo and are 54–60 × 30–35 μm in size. The eggs of *E. boehmi* resemble those of *Trichuris vulpis* and the other capillarids that may be present in canine faecal samples (*Eucoleus aerophilus*, *Pearsonema plica*). Eggs of *E. boehmi* can be differentiated from those of *T. vulpis* based on size and morphology. *Trichuris* eggs are 72–90 × 32–40 μm in size and the shell wall surface is smooth. The bipolar plugs tend to be more prominent and have ridges that give the appearance that they are threaded into the shell wall.

The bipolar plugs of capillarid eggs lack ridges and the shell wall surface has a pattern unique for each of the species. The shell surface pattern of *E. boehmi* consists of fine pitting.

How do you treat E. boehmi?

Treatment using an oral dose of ivermectin at 0.2 mg/kg (this dose is not safe for use in collie-type breeds) appeared to be effective in a naturally infected dog. Similar results were reported using milbemycin oxime (2.0 mg/kg, oral). Failure to control an *E. boehmi* infection in two dogs has been reported using ivermectin (0.2–0.3 mg/kg, oral) and fenbendazole (50 mg/kg, oral, once a day for 10 days).

How do you treat E. aerophilus?

Fenbendazole (30 mg/kg, oral, once a day for 2 days, repeated every 2 weeks for a total of four treatments) was reported to be safe and effective in the treatment of clinically affected arctic foxes. Use of fenbendazole (50 mg/kg, oral, once a day for 14 days) in a dog and abamectin (0.3 mg/kg, subcutaneous, repeated in 2 weeks) in a cat were also reported to be effective treatments for *E. aerophilus* infection. Anthelmintics with apparent efficacy against *E. boehmi* (e.g. ivermectin, milbemycin oxime) may also be useful in cases of *E. aerophilus* infection.

Feline Aelurostrongylosis

What is Aelurostrongylus abstrusus?

This is the only lungworm of domestic cats. *A. abstrusus* occurs in the terminal respiratory bronchioles and alveolar ducts in the lung parenchyma of domestic cats and has a worldwide distribution. In North America it has been reported in Canada and the USA in the east, south-east, south-west, west coast and Hawaii. It is endemic in the UK but prevalence studies are very old and very little is known of the current situation.

How do cats acquire A. abstrusus?

Cats acquire infection by the ingestion of infective third-stage larvae contained in terrestrial gastropod intermediate hosts (slugs, land snails) or a wide range of paratenic hosts (amphibians, reptiles, birds, small rodents). Adult worms are 4–10 mm in length. Mature females produce undifferentiated eggs, which develop and hatch as first-stage larvae before they leave their host. The larvae are coughed up, swallowed and passed in the faeces. The prepatent period is about 5–6 weeks and infected cats shed L1 larvae in the faeces for a period that usually lasts 2–7 months, with a peak in shedding 10–17 weeks after infection. There is a delayed onset of patency, less larval shedding and a more erratic shedding pattern after re-exposure in cats that have been infected previously.

What is the clinical presentation of A. abstrusus?

Infections are usually subclinical. Heavy infections can result in severe and potentially fatal respiratory disease. Clinically affected cats often show signs of cough, dyspnoea and fever and may suffer anorexia and emaciation. As with *C. vulpis* infection in dogs, *A. abstrusus* infection may be misdiagnosed as allergic respiratory disease and show a positive response to administration of corticosteroids and bronchodilators. Infection occurs more often in younger cats (3 months to 3 years) and outdoor cats. Pneumothorax and pyothorax secondary to *A. abstrusus* infection have been reported in a kitten; it has been speculated that third-stage larvae had become contaminated with *Salmonella typhimurium* in the lumen of the intestine and carried it to the lungs.

How do you diagnose A. abstrusus?

Diagnosis is by detection of L1 larvae in faeces (Fig. 3.7), bronchial mucus or pleural fluid. False-negative results in larval detection can occur due to sporadic shedding patterns. Faecal detection occurs by Baermann examination, direct smear and FLOTAC device. The Baermann is considered the most sensitive method for larval detection. The FLOTAC device was

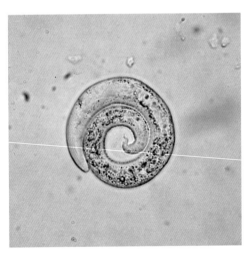

Fig. 3.7. Larva of feline lungworm, *Aelurostrongylus abstrusus*. It has a tail with S-shaped bend and a dorsal spine.

considered more effective in larval recovery than the Baermann technique when compared on samples collected from a single cat infected with *A. abstrusus*. The larvae are 360–400 μm in length and the tail ends in a distinctive sinus wave-shaped kink with a prominent dorsal spine. A nested PCR assay for *A. abstrusus* infection used on Baermann sediment, faeces and pharyngeal swabs has recently been developed in Europe and shows great promise; it had a reported specificity of 100% and sensitivity of 96.6%. Additional diagnostic testing options would involve radiography, transtracheal wash and bronchoalveolar lavage. Radiographic changes tend to show a mixed pattern, with an alveolar pattern predominating during the period of heaviest larval shedding (5–15 weeks post infection) followed by bronchial and interstitial patterns. Computed tomography (CT) images may also be useful in assessing lesions in cats infected with *A. abstrusus*.

How do you treat A. abstrusus?

Options currently available for treating cats infected with *A. abstrusus* include fenbendazole, moxidectin, selamectin, eprinomectin and emodepside. Of these options, fenbendazole and eprinomectin are both licensed for treatment of *A. abstrusus* in the UK. One to two applications of selamectin (6 mg/kg, topical) were reported to be effective in the treatment of one of three cats. Ivermectin (0.4 mg/kg, subcutaneous, repeated in 2 weeks) has been reported to be effective in the treatment of several cats. Fenbendazole (20 mg/kg, oral, once a day for 5 days or 50 mg/kg, oral, once a day for 15 days) was reported to be effective in the treatment of *A. abstrusus* infection in cats. One to three topical applications of moxidectin (1 mg/kg in combination with imidacloprid) appeared to be effective in the treatment of eight cats infected with *A. abstrusus*. Abamectin (0.3 mg/kg, subcutaneous, repeated in 2 weeks) appeared to be effective in the treatment of one cat. Eprinomectin 0.4% w/v in combination with fipronil 8.3% w/v, (S)-methoprene 10% w/v and praziquantel 8.3% w/v in a spot-on solution which are also used to treat ectoparasites and tapeworms has also been demonstrated to be safe and efficacious in treating *A. abstrusus* infection, with faecal larval reductions of 90–91.6%

Lung Fluke Infection

What is Paragonimus kellicotti and where does it occur?

Paragonimus kellicotti is a trematode that occurs in the lung parenchyma infecting dogs, cats, pigs, goats and various wildlife species in endemic areas that include much of the eastern half of North America. Infections are most common in the north-central and south-eastern states of the USA. Faecal examination surveys have indicated a low prevalence of infection

(< 1%); however, these results are likely an underestimate due to suboptimal detection sensitivity of the flotation technique for fluke eggs. Infection with *P. kellicotti* was found to be the cause of disease in 8% (3 of 37) of cats showing signs of chronic respiratory disease in Louisiana. This fluke is not thought to be endemic in the UK.

How does P. kellicotti *live?*

Adult flukes are 10–13 × 4–6 mm in size and occur inside capsules situated in the lung parenchyma; they rarely occur in other tissues. These flukes are easily differentiated from the nematode lungworms of dogs and cats by the body shape and presence of oral and ventral suckers. Capsules are 2–5 cm in diameter with walls 1–4 mm thick; they usually contain two or more flukes and are connected to the bronchioles. Capsules occur most often in the caudal lung lobes (right > left). Eggs passed in faeces that are deposited into water develop and hatch ciliated miracidia, which infect the first intermediate host, aquatic snails (*Pomatiopsis lapidaria*, *Pomatiopsis cincinnatiensis*). Animals acquire infection by the ingestion of metacercaria contained in the tissues of the second intermediate host, crayfish (*Cambarus* spp., *Oronectes* spp.). Prevalence of infection in crayfish can be as high as 94% in a stream in the late summer peak period. In addition, rodents predating on infected crayfish can serve as paratenic hosts. The prepatent period is 5–7 weeks. Infections have been reported to last as long as 4 years.

What are the clinical features of P. kellicotti?

Clinical features include a cough that is sometimes accompanied by sneezing, exercise intolerance, haemoptysis and dyspnoea. Infections can be subclinical to fatal. Subclinical and clinical pneumothorax may develop due to the rupture of the fluke capsule through the pleura, allowing air to pass from the bronchial system to the pleural space. Infected animals may suffer chronic cough for prolonged periods or die acutely, with no history of clinical disease.

How do you diagnose P. kellicotti?

Definitive diagnosis is by detection of the distinctive operculate eggs of *P. kellicotti* in faeces or bronchial mucus. Faecal detection is best achieved through sedimentation. Eggs may be found by faecal flotation; however, detection sensitivity in samples with low levels of eggs is poor. The eggs are 75–118 × 42–67 µm in size, yellow-brown in colour, and have an operculum at one end. The eggs can be differentiated from those of other trematode or pseudophyllidean tapeworms by the thickened ridge in the shell wall highlighting the opercular line. In addition, fluke capsules can be visualized radiographically as multi-loculated cystic structures 2–5 cm in size in dogs. Lesions in cats are smaller and have a greater density.

How do you treat P. kellicotti?

Current treatment options include extra-label usage of albendazole, fenbendazole, or praziquantel. Albendazole (25 mg/kg, oral, twice a day for 14 days), fenbendazole (50 mg/kg, oral, once a day for 10–14 days) and praziquantel (23 mg/kg, oral, three times a day for 3 days) are recommended as effective in the treatment of dogs and cats infected with *P. kellicotti*.

Tongue Worm (Pentastomida) Infection

What are pentastomids?

Phylum Pentastomida shares features with arthropods but is usually regarded as an independent phylum. The pentastomids (tongue worms) are respiratory endoparasites of reptiles, birds and mammals. Adult pentastomids are white and cylindrical or flattened parasites that possess two distinct body regions: an anterior cephalothorax and an abdomen (Fig. 3.8). *Linguatula serrata* is the most common pentastomid of companion animals, with adult parasites living in the upper respiratory tract and nasal passages of cats and dogs. The life cycle can be direct, through cats and dogs ingesting eggs passed in fomites and faeces. Livestock consuming the eggs act as intermediate hosts, with cats and dogs becoming infected through consumption of viscera. Although this parasite is not endemic in the UK, cases are being seen from dogs imported from Romania, where the parasite is present. Diagnosis may be made by finding the eggs in the faeces or respiratory secretions. There is currently no effective treatment for pentastome infections other than surgical removal

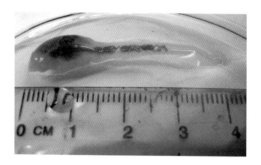

Fig. 3.8. The pentastomid tongue worm, *Linguatula serrata*. (Courtesy of Pedro Serra and Nationwide Labs.)

of the parasites in heavy infections. Humans can act as intermediate hosts through ingestion of eggs, or definitive hosts through consumption of contaminated viscera. In some cases, infected patients develop localized inflammation and such infections are common in the Middle East and Africa where dogs live in very close proximity to livestock.

Self-Assessment Questions

1. **Which of the following is caused by both *Angiostrongylus vasorum* and *Diroifilaria immitis*?**

   (a) Cough

   (b) Coagulopathy

   (c) Congestive heart failure

   (d) Pneumonia

2. **Which of the following is a preventive treatment for *A. vasorum* infection?**

   (a) Monthly moxidectin/imidacloprid spot-on solution

   (b) Oral fenbendazole

   (c) Oral praziquantal

   (d) Oral mebemdazole

3. **Which of the following lungworms has suckers?**

   (a) *Crenosoma vulpis*

   (b) *Oslerus osleri*

   (c) *Aelurostrongylus abstrusus*

   (d) *Paragonimus kellicotti*

4. **_Eucoleus boehmi_ infects which organ tissues?**

   (a) Nasal passages

   (b) Heart

   (c) Liver

   (d) Kidney

5. **Which of the following lungworms is not transmitted by molluscs?**

(a) *Angiostrongylus vasorum*

(b) *Crenosoma vulpis*

(c) *Oslerus osleri*

(d) *Aelurostrongylus abstrusus*

4 Parasites of the Cardiovascular System

Babesiosis

What is babesiosis?

Babesiosis is a blood protozoal disease caused by tick-transmitted intra-erythrocytic protozoa of the genus *Babesia*. These protozoan organisms live inside the red blood cells of animals.

How many Babesia *species infect dogs?*

A number of *Babesia* spp., including *Babesia canis*, *B. gibsoni*, *B. vogelii* and *B. vulpes*, are known to infect dogs in Europe. The two *Babesia* species most commonly infecting dogs are the large piroplasm (*B. canis*) and the small piroplasm (*B. gibsoni*). The former usually occur in pairs and appear pear-shaped, while the latter are smaller and circular.

What is known about the epidemiology of Babesia *infection in the UK?*

Even though babesiosis has been reported in an untravelled British dog, babesiosis has been considered an exotic disease and only identified in dogs returning from travel to Europe. However, in 2016 babesiosis due to *B. canis* was confirmed in four dogs from Essex with no history of foreign travel and *Dermacentor reticulatus* ticks have been incriminated in its transmission. *B. vulpes* has also been isolated from *Ixodes* ticks in the UK.

How do dogs get infected with Babesia?

B. canis is naturally transmitted by *D. reticulatus* ticks, which are found in the UK, and by the brown dog tick *Rhipicephalus sanguineus*, which is common in southern Europe but currently rare in the UK, though it could establish, particularly after the removal of the need for mandatory tick treatment before entry into the UK on 1 January 2012. *R. sanguineus* is the major vector of canine babesiosis in many countries worldwide. A tick typically needs to be attached to a dog for 1–2 days to successfully transmit the infection. Transmission via blood transfusion, transplacental transfer and dog bites has also been reported. *Babesia* organisms can migrate to the tick ovary, leading to transovarial transmission and the maintenance of infection in subsequent generations of ixodid ticks.

What is the clinical presentation of babesiosis?

The clinical course of babesiosis varies from asymptomatic to subclinical to acute, and even fatal outcome. Dogs with clinical babesiosis exhibit anorexia, lethargy, weakness, vomiting, diarrhoea, depression, pale mucous membranes or jaundice. Skin lesions and kidney failure can occur. Pyrexia, splenomegaly, haemolytic anaemia and thrombocytopenia are also clinical findings. Due to the non-specificity of the clinical signs, veterinary staff should ask about history of tick exposure, previous tick treatment and history of travel abroad.

What methods can be used to detect Babesia infection?

Microscopic examination of stained blood smear for characteristic large (*B. canis*) or small (*B. gibsoni*) piroplasms within red blood cells is the easiest, most frequently used and most widely available method for the diagnosis of babesiosis in dogs (Fig. 4.1). Furthermore, the test can be done in-house and is able to diagnose the majority of dogs infected by *B. canis*. However, the sensitivity of this method is lower than that of molecular methods in making a correct diagnosis, especially for small piroplasms, which are hard to observe by light microscopy. For infection with small *Babesia*, more sensitive PCR-based methods are more efficient. Serological tests, such as indirect immunofluorescence antibody test (IFAT) or ELISA, are also available and can allow the determination of the antibody levels, but cannot distinguish among *Babesia* spp. and cannot differentiate between past exposure and current infection. Additionally, false-negatives may occur early in the disease and there could also be cross-reactivity with other species of *Babesia* and apicomplexan protozoa, such as *Toxoplasma gondii* and *Neospora caninum*. The presence of co-infections or concomitant diseases can complicate the diagnosis. In these situations accurate diagnosis is most likely when multiple diagnostic assays, such as microscopic examination and molecular assays, are employed.

What are the treatment and prevention strategies for babesiosis?

Currently, there is no available vaccine for *Babesia* or specific veterinary medicinal product (VMP) authorized in the UK for the treatment of babesiosis

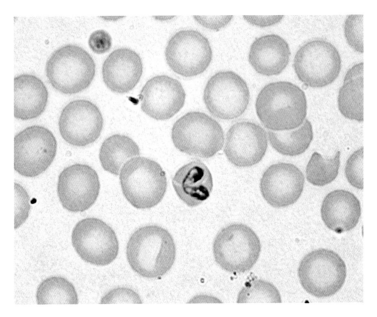

Fig. 4.1. Tick-borne protozoan haemoparasite, *Babesia canis*, in a blood smear.

in dogs. Imizol (Intervet) injection containing imidocarb (85 mg/ml) as imido-carb dipropionate licensed for the treatment of bovine babesiosis can be used off-licence with informed consent (6.6 mg/kg, intramuscular or subcutaneous, given once and repeated in 2–3 weeks). This drug is considered effective for clearance of *B. canis* but is often not effective in clearing smaller *Babesia* species. The safety and effectiveness of imidocarb have not been completely determined in puppies or in breeding, lactating or pregnant animals. Clinical improvement is normally seen within 1–2 days of starting treatment. If this treatment is not suitable for a particular patient, then clinidamycin orally at 12.5 mg/kg twice daily is an alternative with comparable efficacy.

Alternative VMPs can also be imported through the special import scheme. These include imidocarb-containing products similar to Imizol®, such as Carbesia®, which has dogs as a target species and includes dosing infor-mation for dogs. Supportive treatment options, such as blood transfusion, should be considered. It is important to inform dog owners that treatments are unlikely to eliminate the parasite completely, that dogs can become la-tent (long-term) carriers and that these dogs should not be used as blood donors. Also, owners should know that the disease may relapse if such dogs have immunosuppressive therapy or a concurrent illness.

Avoidance of known tick-infested areas, particularly during tick peak seasons, the use of an effective anti-tick medication Collars and daily checking for and removal of ticks as soon as they are discovered may prevent or help to reduce the risk of transmission.

Dirofilariosis (Heartworm, HW Infection)

What are 'heartworms'?

These are worms that live in the heart and are spread from host to host through the bites of mosquitoes. The primary hosts are canids such as dogs, wolves, coyotes and foxes but cats, ferrets and humans can also be infected. They are called filarial worms because they are 'filariaform', i.e. very long and thin. Their first-stage larvae are called microfilariae (mf) and are produced by the adult females. The most important heartworm (HW) is *Dirofilaria immitis*, the males of which measure 12–20 cm and the females 25–31 cm. In general, *D. immitis* is found primarily in the right ventricle and pulmonary arteries of the host and causes respiratory and cardiac diseases. However, heartworms are not always restricted to the cardiorespiratory tract, and immune complex glomerulonephropathy has also been associated with heartworm. Other filarial worms found in dogs are *Dipetalonema* (*Acanthocheilonema*) *reconditum* and *Dirofilaria repens*, which occur in tissues.

How does D. immitis *get into the heart?*

D. immitis has an interesting complex, indirect life cycle, with the dog as definitive host and the mosquito as the intermediate host vector. Female adult worms release microfilariae into the circulatory system, where they can live for up to 2 years. Microfilariae in circulation can be ingested by mosquitoes during a blood meal and develop to infective larval stage (L3) in the stomach of the mosquito. L3s migrate to the mosquito's salivary glands, where they remain until the mosquito feeds on another host and the L3s then move down the mouthparts on to the skin and enter the bite wound into the dog to migrate to the heart. The mosquito (genera *Aedes* and *Culex*) is essential for transmission of the parasite. The prepatent period ranges from 6 to 7 months.

What is the prevalence of heartworm?

Prevalence varies with geographical location but heartworm is widespread throughout North America, southern Europe and some central European countries such as Bulgaria and Romania. Despite improved diagnostic tools, effective preventive measures and increased awareness, heartworm prevalence is increasing in the USA and it is spreading its range in Europe. It is likely that climate change and increased movement of pets and people are driving the spread of the mosquito vector and allowing completion of heartworm life cycles in countries where the climate previously prevented this from occurring.

What pathological injuries can D. immitis cause?

Adults live in the pulmonary arteries of dogs, leading to endothelial damage and myointimal proliferation. Pulmonary artery obstruction causes pulmonary hypertension and thrombosis.

What clinical signs can a dog with heartworm infection exhibit?

Severity of disease and damage to the dogs by heartworm are directly related to the number of adult worms, duration of infection and host response. Infection with *D. immitis* causes multiple organ system dysfunctions, including pulmonary circulation, heart, liver and kidneys. Clinical signs range from being asymptomatic to heart failure. Infected dogs may show exercise intolerance, decreased appetite, loss of weight, cough and listlessness. Animals with severe heartworm disease will show lack of endurance during exercise and in rare situations they may die of sudden heart failure.

What are the clinical stages of heartworm infection?

According to the severity of clinical signs, the diseases can be categorized into three phases: mild to moderate; moderate to severe; and severe (Table 4.1).

What methods are commonly used to detect heartworm?

Diagnosis of heartworm depends on obtaining an accurate patient history, recognition of clinical manifestations and use of several diagnostic procedures. Given that each of the following diagnostic techniques has shortcomings, their use in combination is required to optimize diagnostic accuracy.

Table 4.1. Clinical diagnostic features of stages of heartworm disease

Phase(s)	Clinical features
Mild to moderate	Chronic cough, decreased tolerance towards exercise, dyspnoea (difficult breathing), weight loss, pulmonary changes on thoracic radiography, packed cell volume (PCV) between 20 and 25.
Moderate to severe	Cachexia, exercise intolerance, fainting (syncope), tachycardia, ascites indicates right-sided heart failure, hepatomegaly, pulmonary and cardiac changes on thoracic radiography, PCV < 20.
Severe	Coughing up blood (haemoptysis) indicates severe pulmonary thromboembolism complications; congestive heart failure and vena caval syndrome occur when vena cava is obstructed by adult worms; globinuria due to acute haemolytic shock.

- Complete blood count:
  - anaemia (mild in phase II, severe in phase III);
  - combined eosinophilia and basophilia;
  - leucocytosis and thrombocytopenia associated with thromboembolism.
- Serum biochemical profile and urinalysis:
  - hyperglobulinaemia;
  - proteinuria (common in dogs with severe and chronic infection and may be caused by immune-complex glomerulonephritis or amyloidosis);
  - haemoglobinuria (caused by acute haemolytic crisis during vena cava syndrome).
- Heartworm antigen tests are specific, sensitive serological tests in dogs, which identify adult female *D. immitis* antigen. Antigen tests take 7 months after infection to develop a positive status, thus are not used in testing puppies less than 7 months old.
- Microfilaria identification tests, including the modified Knott's test, filter tests and direct smear. A blood smear may reveal *D. immitis* microfilariae in a dog with heartworm disease but, due to intermittent low circulating numbers, direct smears are insensitive tests for detection.
- Thoracic radiological examination is performed not only as a diagnostic aid but also to predict stage of infection and extent of thromboembolism. Thoracic radiological examination also allows comparison between radiographs taken during treatment and recovery. Thoracic radiographic signs include:
  - enlargement of the main pulmonary artery;
  - lobar arterial enlargement and tortuosity varying from absent (phase I) to severe (phase III);
  - parenchymal lung infiltrates of variable severity which may extend into most or all of one or multiple lung lobes when thromboembolism occurs; and
  - allergic reaction to microfilariae inducing diffuse, symmetrical, alveolar and interstitial infiltrates.
- Echocardiogram may show right ventricular dilation and wall hypertrophy; parallel linear echodensities produced by the worms may be detected in the right ventricle, right atrium and pulmonary artery.
- Electrocardiogram, usually unremarkable, may reflect right ventricle hypertrophy in dogs with severe infection; heart rhythm disturbances rarely seen but may include atrial fibrillation, especially in severe infection.

What is the differential diagnosis of heartworm?

Heartworm must be differentiated from: (i) other causes of pulmonary hypertension and thrombosis, such as hyperadrenocorticism; (ii) other causes of pulmonary disease, including allergic lung disease, chronic obstructive pulmonary disease (COPD), neoplasia, parasitic lung disease, foreign body, pneumonia; and (iii) other causes of ascites, including dilated cardiomyopathy, hypoproteinaemia, hepatic disease, caudal caval or portal vein thromboembolism, neoplasia, pericardial effusion. Thoracic radiological examination and heartworm antigen tests should differentiate all these conditions from heartworm disease.

How can heartworm disease be prevented?

Chemoprophylaxis is nearly 100% effective in preventing heartworm infection when administered appropriately. Several drugs are available. Macrocyclic lactone (ML) derivatives (i.e. ivermectin, milbemycin oxime, moxidectin, selamectin, eprinomectin) are the drugs of choice for chemoprophylaxis in dogs and cats. Moxidectin is licensed for heartworm prophylaxis in ferrets. All the chemoprophylaxis medications are microfilaricidal when administered continuously over a period of time. They should only be administered in endemic countries once antigen testing has been performed to rule out adult heartworm infection. Use of MLs in patients with heartworm infection may lead to anaphylactic complications. Wearing insecticide-impregnated collars (e.g. permethrin) for dogs affords good protection against biting flies like mosquitoes and sandflies (vector of *Leishmania*).

What is 'vena caval syndrome'?

Caval syndrome is a severe complication of heartworm disease in dogs associated with the presence of a large number of worms in the right ventricle (RV), the right atrium (RA) and the vena cava (VC). Tangled masses of worms in the VC and RA interfere with blood return and disrupt the tricuspid valve apparatus, causing tricuspid regurgitation. The syndrome is characterized by acute onset of anorexia, lethargy, weakness, respiratory distress and dark red urine. Clinical signs result from cardiogenic shock, intravascular haemolysis and right heart failure.

How do you treat a dog with heartworm?

The conventional approach is to kill all adult parasites first with an adulticide drug and then all circulating microfilariae with a microfilaricide. Some patients may need hospitalization during adulticide treatment, since severe post-treatment complications are likely. When the adult parasites die, the pulmonary arteries carry them to the lungs, where they eventually decay and are removed by the immune system. Although the adulticide drugs are designed to be slow acting and prevent the accumulation of dead worms all at once in the animal's lungs, the load on the lungs is still immense and stressful to the treated animals. Restriction of activity is required for 4–6 weeks after adulticide administration, especially for severe disease. Hospitalization and cage confinement for a week is recommended for dogs experiencing pulmonary thromboembolic complications.

Approximately 4 weeks following adulticide therapy, microfilaricide treatment should be initiated. This allows enough time for the dog to recover from any injuries associated with HW death. In dogs with severe disease and congestive heart failure, the latter should be treated until the dog becomes stable before administering adulticides. Also, pulmonary failure should be stabilized with antithrombotic agents (e.g. aspirin or heparin) and anti-inflammatory doses of corticosteroid; the case should be monitored using clinical and radiographic parameters. Dogs with vena caval syndrome require surgical removal of adult worms from the right side of the heart and pulmonary artery via the jugular vein by using fluoroscopy and long, flexible alligator forceps. Recent research studies proposed the concept of 'tetracycline *Wolbachia* treatment of heartworms'. This hypothesis is believed to be attributable to clearance of *Wolbachia* (intracellular rickettsial-like organisms found within filarial worms) by tetracycline treatment.

How do you treat a dog with vena caval syndrome?

Treatment includes: (i) administration of oxygen to relieve the hypoxaemia caused by poor cardiac output; (ii) intravenous fluid administration to support circulation; (iii) blood transfusion to stabilize the patient prior to worm removal; (iv) anti-inflammatory doses of glucocorticosteroids and heparin prior to worm removal, because of the risks of antigen release and anaphylactic reaction (associated with worm maceration) and thromboembolism; and (v) surgical worm removal via jugular venotomy with the use of long (20–40 cm), small-diameter, flexible alligator forceps, preferably using echocardiographic or fluoroscopic guidance. Owners should be advised that prognosis is guarded to poor, with a mortality rate of 30–40%, and that strict rest must be enforced.

How is heartworm disease in cats different from dogs?

Although the life cycle of *D. immitis* in cats is similar to that in dogs, feline heartworm infection differs from canine heartworm in a number of characteristics.

- Cats are more resistant to heartworms than dogs.
- The cat does not serve well as a definitive host because of the low microfilaraemias.

- Aberrant migration of fourth-stage larvae (L4) occurs more frequently in cats than in dogs and ectopic heartworms have been found in the body cavities and central nervous systems of infected cats.
- There are fewer adult worms in feline infection (usually fewer than six).
- The lifespan of the adult worms is only about half the length of that in dogs (2–3 years compared with 5–7 years).
- The average prepatent period is 7–8 months (1–2 months longer than that in dogs).
- Heartworm rarely reaches the adult stage in cats.
- Heartworm infection in cats is often self-limiting (infected cats are frequently managed with supportive treatment).
- The overall prevalence in cats is between 5% and 10% of that in dogs.

What signs do you expect to see if a cat has heartworm disease?

Signs include tachypnoea, dyspnoea, increased breathing sounds and coughing; also right-sided heart murmur if worms disrupt the tricuspid valve. Gastrointestinal signs, such as vomiting, can be seen. Rarely, syncope, neurological signs, embolic events and caval syndrome are reported. Clinical signs are most likely to manifest in cats during initial worm migration into the pulmonary arteries or at the time of death of the worms. Cats tend to have more lung damage than dogs, because worms die faster in cats. Sudden death occurs due to acute respiratory failure from pulmonary thromboembolism. Chronic respiratory disease caused by heartworm infections in cats is known as heartworm-associated respiratory disease (HARD).

Why is diagnosis of heartworm disease in cats challenging?

False-negatives are common in cats due to low worm burdens, light antigen load, all-male infection and the fact that cats are rarely microfilaraemic (i.e. blood evaluation for larvae is very insensitive). Therefore, a thorough diagnostic approach using a combination of chest radiographs, serology (for both antibody and antigen) and echocardiography is necessary. Necropsy confirmation of heartworm disease is the 'gold standard' but in the living patient positive serology in combination with clinical signs is often relied upon, with ultrasound to rule out the presence of adult worms.

What are the public health implications of heartworm?

In general, cases of human infection are rare and heartworms represent no serious zoonotic potential. In some cases, heartworms were found to induce benign pulmonary nodules that can be radiographically confused with cancer. Until 1999, most human cases in Europe originated from Italy,

France, Greece and Spain but autochthonous cases are now regularly reported from central and northern Europe. The worms do not develop to adults in humans.

How do you treat a cat with heartworm?

Treatment of adult heartworm infection is very difficult in cats, with a higher risk of thromboembolism. Cats with mild signs may resolve the infection on their own. Microfilaricide treatment is usually unnecessary, since cats have few circulating microfilariae. Surgical treatment, where adult worms are physically removed from the heart, is indicated in cats that develop vena cava syndrome. Bronchitic signs may require steroids; and oxygen, intravenous fluids and bronchodilators such as the xanthines or terbutaline are all useful in helping to stabilize acute patients, particularly those in respiratory distress. Experts recommend taking preventive measures in areas where the prevalence of canine heartworm is high. A number of safe and effective macrocyclic lactone drugs are available for prophylaxis in cats. Monthly macrocyclic lactones such as selamectin, ivermectin, moxidectin, eprinomectin and milbemycin are considered safe and effective.

How do you distinguish between microfilariae of Dirofilaria immitis and Dipetalonema (Acanthocheilonema) reconditum?

Dipetalonema reconditum males are 9–17 mm long and the females are 20–32 mm long. *Dirofilaria repens* and *D. reconditum* live in subcutaneous tissue and are of limited veterinary importance, but cause lesions in cutaneous tissues due to Microfilariae (mf) of *Dipetalonema (Acanthocheilonema) reconditum*. In dogs the most common species of filariae are *D. immitis*, *D. repens* and *D. reconditum*. Infection can be diagnosed through morphological observation (how they differ) of circulating mf, detection of circulating antigens (*D. immitis* only), histochemical or immunohistochemical staining of circulating mf or through molecular approaches. *D. reconditum* mf should be differentiated from *D. immitis* (cause of heartworm disease) mf because their occurrence often overlaps in the same endemic area (see below).

How do dogs acquire Dipetalonema reconditum?

Adult nematodes live in the subcutaneous tissues, kidneys and body cavity of dogs and other canids. Fertilized females shed larvae/mf, which migrate into the bloodstream. Fleas, the brown dog tick, the dog sucking louse and the dog biting louse act as intermediate hosts for *D. reconditum*. Following ingestion of an infected blood meal by the intermediate host, mf develop to the infective stage in about 1–2 weeks and then migrate to the head of the insect. The mf pass to the dog when the infected arthropod feeds on the next host.

Is it clinically significant?

Yes, because of the close morphological similarity of *D. reconditum* mf to those of *D. immitis*, which may lead to misdiagnosis, especially in heartworm-endemic areas. Several other *Dipetalonema* species and *D. repens* affect humans. Treatment is not normally indicated, because this parasite is not usually considered pathogenic. However, the presence of adult worms may occasionally cause subcutaneous ulceration and abscessation.

Self-Assessment Questions

1. *Dirofilaria immitis* is found primarily in which chamber of the heart?

(a) Left atrium

(b) Left ventricle

(c) Right atrium

(d) Right ventricle

2. What is the vector for *D. immitis*?

(a) Slugs and snails

(b) Mosquito

(c) Sand fly

(d) Ticks

3. What is the lifespan of adult *D. immitis* worms in dogs?

(a) 2–3 months

(b) 5–7 months

(c) 2–3 years

(d) 5–7 years

4. What is the lifespan of adult *D. immitis* worms in cats?

(a) 2–3 months

(b) 5–7 months

(c) 2–3 years

(d) 5–7 years

5. **What is the average prepatent period of *D. immitis* in cats?**

(a) 7–8 weeks

(b) 9–12 weeks

(c) 7–8 months

(d) 9–12 months

5 Parasites of the Skin and Muscles

Flea Infestations

What are fleas and how do they thrive?

Fleas are obligate blood-sucking insects, which have evolved to live in close proximity to their hosts and the host habitat. In the case of cat fleas and to some extent dog fleas, this adaptation causes severe domestic household infestations. Adult fleas seen on pets are glossy brown/black in colour, flattened from side to side, and are equipped with very powerful back legs for jumping. They have a set of combs at the junction of the head and thorax (pronotal ctenidia) and another set near the mouthparts (genal ctenidia). This morphology varies in different species (rabbit fleas, rodent and bird fleas, for example, which may occasionally be found on cats and dogs) and flea species identification can be important in control programmes advised for flea-infested households. Cat and dog fleas may cause intense itching and induce allergic reactions in susceptible animals and they also bite pet owners.

Flea infestations are probably the most common ectoparasites of dogs and cats. Although more than 2200 species and subspecies of fleas are known throughout the world, the cat flea *Ctenocephalides felis* (Fig. 5.1a) remains the dominant species on domestic pets. That said, rabbit fleas, while not persistently residing on the pet, are seen regularly in practice, as are infestations of household bird fleas. These incidents are possibly more common now than dog flea infestations, which have become quite rare.

Understanding their unique life cycle (and explaining this to clients) is very important before initiating control. Cat and dog fleas produce lots of eggs while on the pet and as these are shaken off they may be widely distributed in the household environment. There they develop into larvae, which feed on dried dirt originating from adult fleas (excess regurgitated blood) and other detritus. In the infested domestic setting, the accumulated larval offspring develop over time into new adults and thereby continuously infest and reinfest pets. Furthermore, the final 'chrysalis' stage or pupa (Fig. 5.1b) is sticky and becomes surrounded by debris; in this way it is protected and is resistant to treatments applied to carpets and bedding. Once the pupa has fully developed, the immature or 'pharate' adult flea within the cocoon can be stimulated to emerge from the cocoon by vibrations, carbon dioxide and heat.

Can fleas survive for long periods?

The entire life cycle of C. *felis* can be completed in 12–14 days, or it can be prolonged up to a year or more: if the pre-emerged adult does not receive an emergence stimulus, it may remain quiescent in the cocoon (Fig. 5.1c) until a suitable host arrives and pupae have been recorded as lying dormant for up to 2 years until favourable conditions occur. However, under most occupied household conditions, nearly all cat fleas will complete their life cycle within 3–8 weeks. As with immature life stages, survival of adult fleas is highly dependent on temperature and humidity.

One study has shown that, in moisture-saturated air, 62% of adult C. *felis* survived for 62 days, whereas only 5% survived for 12 days when maintained at 22.5°C and 60% relative humidity (RH). It is unlikely that adult or immature fleas in the premises can survive during winter in northern temperate regions. It has also been shown that no life cycle stage (egg, larva, pupa, or adult) can survive for 10 days at 3°C (37.4°F) or 5 days at 1°C.

Where do fleas hide and when are they a problem?

It is important to realize that any adult fleas seen on a pet represent the 'tip of the iceberg' and that large numbers of immature fleas are likely be

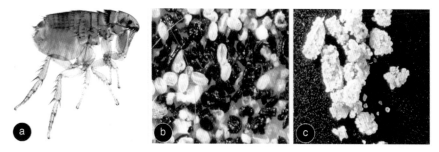

Fig. 5.1. (a) Cat flea, *Ctenocephalides felis*. Flea mouthparts are adapted for sucking blood. In cat flea, the first two cheek comb spines are about the same length, whereas in dog flea, *Ctenocephalides canis*, the front-most spine of the cheek comb is shorter than the second spine. (b) Flea pupa. (c) Flea cocoon.

undergoing covert development, sometimes well away from the pet. Newly emerged fleas, in carpets or from outdoors, will bite most animals, including humans, if their preferred host is scarce, though they will not persistently infest humans. Because C. *felis* is not highly cold tolerant, it has been postulated that in cold climates it survives in the urban environment, as adults on untreated dogs and cats or on small wild mammals. Once on a host, C. *felis* initiates feeding within seconds to minutes. In one study, approximately 25% of fleas were blood-fed within 5 min; and in another, the volume of blood consumed by fleas was quantifiable within 5 min. Mating occurs on the host after feeding and can occur within 8–24 h.

When fleas that have been on a host for several days are removed, they die within 1–4 days. Experimental work has shown that when cats are allowed to groom freely, they will ingest or groom off a substantial number of fleas in a few days. When cat fleas were allowed to feed for only 12 h and then removed from their host, 5% were still alive at 14 days. This is of particular importance, because one study showed that when cats were housed adjacent to each other but physically separated, 3–8% of the fleas moved from one cat to another. However, when cats were housed in the same cage, 2–15% of the fleas transferred. Therefore, it is possible for a few adult fleas to transfer from one host to another but it is far more likely that most flea infestations originate from previously unfed fleas emerging from environments that have supported development of immature life stages.

C. *felis* is referred to as the cat flea because it was first described from a cat, but it is actually able to infest approximately 50 species of animals. Cat fleas exhibit an extremely prolific reproduction and, as a result, environmental infestation is difficult to control, taking a minimum of 90 days to eliminate indoor infestations. If outdoors (e.g. inside kennels), there are additional problems. An infestation in the home may not be obvious until the third generation of fleas has developed.

What are the differential diagnoses for flea infestation and how can a flea infestation be confirmed?

The most likely differential diagnosis for C. *felis* (cat flea) infestation includes *Sarcoptes scabiei* (scabies mites), *Otodectes cynotis* (ear mite) in severe infestions, *Trichodectes canis* (lice), *Cheyletiella yasguri* (dog fur mite, or 'walking dandruff'), dermatitis secondary to infection or allergic skin disease such as atopy. A coat brushing with a flea comb or adhesive tape impressions will reveal flea dirt as black specks, flea eggs as white specks, or adult fleas. Viewing these findings under the microscope will confirm flea life stages. Also, a wet paper will turn red due to the blood content in the flea faeces if combings are placed on the surface. To investigate other causes of pruritis, such as mange mites, repeated skin scrapes will be required to examine for the burrowing species *S. scabiei*, which can be difficult to reveal. An aural swab may be used to make a smear to be viewed microscopically for *O. cynotis*, which may have spread to the body, and for bacteria and yeast. If the owner has developed pruritic skin lesions, as happens with flea bites, other ectoparasites have to be excluded. If lesions are most often seen on the arms where the pet has been held, this could be due to *Cheyletiella* spp. or *Sarcoptes*, both of which are zoonotic, with the latter a cause of serious mange in dogs but very rarely associated with cats. If the owner has a history of a series of bites around the ankles, this indicates that the infestation is coming from inside the home – from carpets, for example. Bites around the waist indicate flea pupae hatching from the couch or other soft furnishings when the owner is seated. Some people are less sensitive to bites than others, so if the owners have not noticed bites, this does not rule out an internal infestation.

What kind of diseases can fleas transmit?

Flea-borne bacterial infections Fleas serve as the vector of microbial agents, some of which may affect humans. *Bartonella henselae* is the causative agent of cat scratch disease (CSD) and can cause flu-like symptoms in humans and bacillary angiomatosis in immunodeficient patients. Other blood-borne pathogens that have been isolated from fleas include *Rickettsia felis* (agent of cat-flea rickettsioses) and *Haemoplasma* spp., which cause anaemia in cats. Rodent fleas can also transmit bubonic plague (*Yersinia pestis*) and murine (endemic) typhus (*Rickettsia typhi*).

Flea-borne intestinal helminthiasis *Ctenocephalides* fleas act as the intermediate hosts for the tapeworm of dogs and cats, *Dipylidium caninum*. Adult *D. caninum* excrete gravid proglottids (containing packets of eggs) in the environment, on which flea larvae feed. *D. caninum* larvae then hatch and migrate into the body of the flea larvae; and following metamorphosis, the infective cysticercoid stage is present in the adult flea. Dogs or cats become infected when they self-groom and ingest infected adult fleas (i.e. containing cysticercoid). Animals infected with *D. caninum* may have up to 130 adult tapeworms, because larval fleas can ingest whole worm packets, resulting in the development of multiple cysticercoids per flea, and each cysticercoid will lead to the development of an adult tapeworm. Hence, it is essential to control fleas in order to prevent *D. caninum* infection in dogs and cats. In rare cases, *D. caninum* can also affect humans, particularly children. Fleas can also act as the intermediate host of *Hymenolepis nana* and the non-pathogenic subcutaneous filarid nematode of dogs, *Acanthocheilonema (Dipetalonema) reconditum*.

What is flea allergy dermatitis?

Flea allergy dermatitis (FAD) is the most common dermatological disease of dogs and a major cause of feline miliary dermatitis. It is an immunological disease in which a hypersensitive state is produced in a host, resulting from the injection of antigenic material from the salivary glands of fleas. The way in which an animal responds to FAD varies between species; for example, cats typically develop military dermatitis. In dogs, the dermatitis is typically confined to the dorsal lumbosacral area (Fig. 5.2).

What flea control questions and problems might face a veterinary nurse?

Firstly, armed with the above knowledge, a nurse must introduce concepts of integrated control. Integrated flea control consists of four steps to break the flea life cycle at as many stages as possible:

1. Using a licensed product on the pet that is fully effective against adult fleas (an 'adulticide') and kills fleas before they can produce eggs (the reproductive breakpoint).
2. Using an insect growth regulator (explained below), either directly into the environment or on the pet to break the flea life cycle.
3. Mechanical measures such as washing bedding to at least 60°C and daily vacuuming to reduce organic matter on which flea larvae feed, as well as physically removing pupae from the environment.
4. Education – ensuring that the client is aware of the importance of the above steps and treatment timeframes, so that client expectations of success in eliminating fleas from the household are realistic.

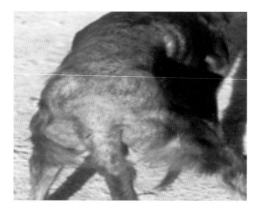

Fig. 5.2. A dog showing the classical skin lesion of flea allergy dermatitis.

Integrated control also involves making a decision about the choice of a product that will prevent other ectoparasitic infestations besides fleas, such as ticks.

How do insect growth regulators work?

Insect growth regulators (IGRs) are available for flea control. They act to inhibit insect development into the next immature life stage. For instance, they may inhibit insect chitin synthesis (a protein needed to build the insect's larval and egg cuticle) (e.g. lufenuron). Other types mimic juvenile growth hormone levels, which would normally drop to initiate the next life stage (e.g. s-methoprene).

In the case of a premises infestation, the IGRs in the flea environment will prevent viable eggs accumulating and hatching and will prevent larvae developing into pupae. However, there are no products available that effectively kill the pupal stage, because these are buried deep in the pile of the carpet, in cracks and crevices of the floor or within soft furnishings and are protected by their cocoons, which are further inaccessible, being covered in debris.

What advice do you give to a client whose pet is heavily infested?

The client's household is likely to have an established infestation rather than, say, an externally acquired transient problem. Firstly, all pets in the household must be treated, with an approved licensed product that kills adult fleas within 24 h or less. Untreated pets must not be allowed access to the premises. In addition, all areas of the home/car/shed/caravan that the pet frequents, especially for sleeping, should ideally be treated with an IGR to help break the flea life cycle and hence reduce the time it takes to clear the infestation. Treated pets should be allowed access to all areas where they have previously been allowed as newly emerged hungry fleas will then be exposed. Owners need to be aware that pupae will continue to be a source of new fleas for at least the next 2–3months until this reservoir is naturally depleted. Advice given should include the principles of integrated control and must necessarily be tailored to suit individual situations.

During a household flea infestation, a client changes to a different flea product due to efficacy concerns and this second product appears to be effective. How might this be explained?

There are no insecticides that kill flea pupae. The so-called 'pupal window' period is the time it takes for fleas to hatch from pupae already in the household, which is usually 2–3 months but can be much longer, depending on temperature, relative humidity and availability of hosts for new fleas. Pupae can lie dormant for up to 2 years if left undisturbed in cool climates. If clients have not been informed about this 'flea reservoir' they will typically get very frustrated with whichever product they were first dispensing and may choose to swap products. By the time this happens, the pupal window may have been coming towards its natural end and the infestation was clearing anyway. It is therefore advisable to pick a licensed product and keep using it at recommended intervals until the infestation comes to an end and then continue to use preventive treatments all year round.

Why might flea control fail?

Possible explanations for failure include that the dog and cat may not have received the topical adulticide application at the recommended treatment intervals. There may be untreated animals in the home or otherwise in contact, or the pet has been washed with a shampoo while using a spot-on product that is not absorbed systemically. The presence of adult cat fleas despite use of effective adulticide treatment may be due to a lack of compliance or the insecticide may not have been administered correctly. Resistance to flea products in the domestic setting has never been documented.

Fly Strike

What is fly strike in rabbits?

During the summer months, emergency clinics see a considerable increase in the number of fly strike cases in pet rabbits. Fly strike is a devastating condition caused by the fly *Lucilia sericata*, or green bottle fly, the same species that causes the common fly strike problem in sheep. These flies are attracted to damp fur soiled with urine or soft faeces. Each fly can lay up to 200 eggs on the skin at the rear end of an animal, which within hours, hatch into maggots and grow by feeding on the flesh of the rabbit. The maggots can very quickly eat away large areas of tissue around the bottom, tail, scent glands, belly and back and affected rabbits are quite literally 'eaten alive'.

What are the symptoms of fly strike?

Initially, the pet may seem quiet, so it is important to check the rabbit's fur daily for any signs of maggots. As the maggots grow and eat away more surface area of the skin, severe shock develops, eventually leading to collapse and death.

How do you treat fly strike?

If veterinary help is sought early, the patient can be saved by receiving prompt treatment comprising the removal of every single maggot (especially the small ones and looking for any unhatched eggs), clipping and cleaning debris from the fur, pain relief, topical soothing products and antibiotics. Fluid therapy, treatment of gastrointestinal complications and syringe feeding may be required in more severe cases. If extensive tissue loss has occurred a rabbit may need to be euthanized to relieve suffering.

What can be done to prevent fly strike?

Many affected rabbits are very well looked after in general but it only takes a small amount of soiling for the flies to strike. Rabbits that cannot groom themselves effectively due to long fur, obesity, arthritis or painful teeth are at greater risk. Checking the rabbit's bottom daily will help to detect infestation early. Topical products containing the IGR cyromazine are also effective to prevent fly eggs from hatching. After an application, protection lasts for up to 8–10 weeks.

Louse Infestations

What are lice?

Lice are wingless insects, flattened from top to bottom, that cling to hair or feathers of animals by means of their strong claws. Lice species can be distinguished by the characteristic shape and width of their heads and there are two types, with a similar life cycle. Biting lice can generally be distinguished from sucking lice by the flattened, wide head. Sucking lice tend to have longer pointed heads and mouthparts. Biting or chewing lice belong to the order Mallophaga and feed mostly on skin debris and secretions. Those that belong to the order Anoplura feed differently – they suck blood.

Female lice lay white eggs with lids ('nits') on the animal's fur (Fig. 5.3a), sticking each one firmly to a hair shaft. Nymphs hatch from the eggs, feeding and undergoing three moults before becoming adults. The life cycle can be completed in 14–21 days. Transfer of lice between hosts is mainly through close physical contact between animals. The term 'pediculosis' is used for

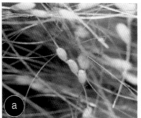
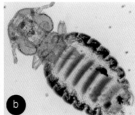
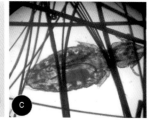

Fig. 5.3. (**a**) Louse egg 'nit'. (**b**) Canine chewing/biting louse, *Trichodectes canis*. This louse is about 1.5 mm long, with body flattened top to bottom and a broad, round head. (**c**) Chewing louse of cats, *Felicola subrostratus*, readily identified by the unique shape of its head.

disease due to severe infestations, often associated with older animals unable to groom, those in general poor condition or those suffering from neglect.

Which types of lice infest dogs and cats and how do they cause harm?

Dogs may be infested with two species: the blood sucking louse *Linognathus setosus* and the chewing/biting species *Trichodectes canis* (Fig. 5.3b). Cats are infested with only one louse species, *Felicola subrostratus*, a chewing type (Fig. 5.3c). *T. canis* is the most common species on dogs; the lice are 1–2 mm in length, yellowish, and dorsoventrally flattened with a clearly recognizable round head, which is the same width as the abdomen. They attach to hair shafts typically around the head, neck, back and tail area, where they feed on dermal debris and exudates from skin lesions. Mature females lay several eggs per day and the nymphs, which resemble the adults, hatch from the eggs within 1–2 weeks of oviposition. Adults live for about 1 month and are very mobile, producing intense irritation, pruritus and scratching.

Linognathus lice are much less common. They are brownish-yellow, measuring 1.5–1.7 mm; the head is long, narrow and pointed, significantly narrower than the slender and elongated abdomen. These lice feed on blood, with females laying one egg per day. Sucking lice infestations are most commonly found on long-haired breeds, such as spaniels, basset hounds and Afghan hounds. Preferred sites for these lice include the ears, neck and back. The infestations may result in pruritus, alopecia and excoriations and severely infested dogs may become anaemic.

F. subrostratus (the biting louse of cats) are yellow to beige and measure 1–1.5 mm. They have a distinctive triangular-shaped head and mouthparts with a median longitudinal groove to grasp an individual hair. Infestations most commonly occur on the face, back and pinnae. Long-haired breeds are more prone to severe infestations, especially under matted or neglected fur. Lice infestations in cats may result in dull and ruffled hair, scaling, crusts, alopecia and significant skin irritation leading to pruritus, dermatitis, excoriation and alopecia with broken hair shafts.

Can owners become infested from their pets?

No. Lice are species specific and so people do not become infested by lice from their pets.

How do you diagnose suspected louse infestations?

Close observation, brushings, hair plucks and adhesive tape strips may reveal adult lice and lice eggs attached to hairs. All these stages are visible to the naked eye but microscopic examination will confirm their presence.

What are the general considerations for louse control?

Lice infestations are frequently encountered in neglected animals, for example those subjected to overcrowding, poor sanitation or with underlying health conditions which predispose to growth of louse populations. Most healthy animals are able to tolerate lice in low numbers. When spotted, lice can be easily killed and traditional treatments have included the use of conventional insecticidal shampoos, sprays and powders. Biting and sucking lice infestations on dogs have been eliminated following a single topical spot-on application with 9.1% wt/wt imidacloprid. Biting lice infestations on dogs have been successfully treated following a single topical spot-on application with 10% imidacloprid + 2.5% moxidectin, 10% fipronil, or 65% permethrin. Biting lice on cats and dogs have been successfully treated with a single topical spot-on application of selamectin. Transmission is through close contact and so pets of the same or closely associated species should all be treated to avoid spread. Because there is no persistent environmental stage, lice infestations can be controlled by physical removal of lice and eggs with a nit comb. However, cats and dogs have a much greater surface area of hair compared with treating human head lice by this method and combing may unintentionally aid in the spread of the parasite if combs are not thoroughly cleaned and all lice life stages destroyed.

Do owners need to treat the environment if their pets have lice?

Although there is no persistent environmental stage and the whole life cycle takes place on the pet, lice can survive in the environment for 1–2 days. If multiple pets are in a household, it is therefore worth treating bedding with a pyrethroid spray or washing at more than 60°C. It is not essential to treat the environment as long as all in-contact pets of the same species are being treated.

Is there any evidence of resistance in lice to insecticides?

Human head and body lice insecticide resistance is well documented and intensive treatment along with the lack of wildlife reservoir hosts (refugia) has led to widespread resistance to conventional insecticides. However, this has not been the case in cat and dog lice.

Mite Infestations and Mange

What are mites and what is mange?

Mites are small parasitic arthropods of birds and domesticated and wild animals. They are not insects, but acarines, which are in the same class as ticks. Morphologically, therefore, parasitic mites do not have distinct body regions (as do insects) and the head and thorax are fused together, as in ticks. Mites that cause skin conditions in dogs and cats (this has the special name, mange) are small and soft bodied and examples are *Sarcoptes* spp., *Notoedres cati* and *Demodex* spp. These types actually tunnel into the skin or hair follicles to lay eggs and are known as 'burrowing mites'. There are others that feed on the skin surface and are described as 'non-burrowing'; the dandruff mite, *Cheyletiella* spp., and the ear mite, *Otodectes* spp., are examples of the latter. They feed superficially on skin and scales. Identification of mites is based on the morphology of the adults and detection generally requires skin repeat scrapings. *Demodex* is an exceptional mite in that it lives in the hair follicles and sebaceous glands, and in cats and dogs causes demodectic mange in susceptible animals.

Cheyletiella, the 'walking dandruff' mite

What are Cheyletiella *mites and how do they complete their life cycle?*

Cheyletiella spp. (Fig. 5.4) are non-burrowing and live in the keratin layer of the epidermis, consuming surface debris and tissue fluids. The eggs are attached to the host animal's hair and are smaller than the average louse egg or 'nit'. Three morphologically similar species of *Cheyletiella* exist: *C. yasguri* in dogs, *C. blakei* in cats and *C. parasitivorax* in rabbits. Adult mites are rather large with an ovoid shape, measuring about 400 µm in length, with characteristic curved palpal claws at the head end. They move rapidly and induce bran-like exfoliative debris on the rumps and backs of animals, resulting in a 'walking dandruff' appearance (the colloquial name for the skin condition these mites cause). They do not burrow but pierce

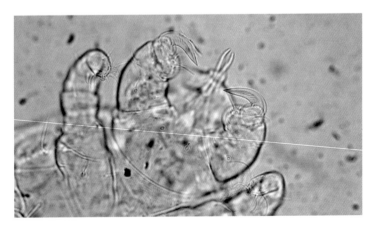

Fig. 5.4. *Cheyletiella*, surface-dwelling (non-burrowing) mite. This mite resides in the keratin layer of the skin and in the hair coat of the host. It is referred to as 'walking dandruff' because *Cheyletiella* mites often resemble large, mobile flakes of dandruff.

the skin with stylet-like chelicerae to feed on lymph. The pre-larva, and larva, develop within the egg and moult through two nymphal stages before becoming adults. Young animals, especially when housed in cages or kennels, and debilitated individuals are particularly susceptible to infestation. Heavily infested dogs may have excessive shedding of hair, inflammation and hyperaesthesia of the dorsal skin. Cats are primarily affected around the head and trunk.

What are the clinical features of cheyletiellosis and differential diagnosis?

These are pruritus and excessive dorsal scaling, and ceruminous otitis externa. Flea infestation, otodectic mange and scabies should also be considered as a cause; less likely differentials include pediculosis, primary seborrhoea, malnutrition and demodicosis.

Which diagnostic tests can confirm cheyletiellosis?

It is best to examine debris from a coat brushing, preferably on to a dark surface, using a hand lens and examining the debris for movement. Low-power microscopic examination of superficial skin scrapings in liquid paraffin or acetate tape preparations from the skin surface may allow detection and identification of the mite, and the technique can cover large areas and improve sensitivity.

Can owners become infested?

Yes, all three species can cause a transient problem in humans, manifesting as papular lesions. A history of a recently introduced pet in the household may be a clue to the diagnosis. Infested pets may be asymptomatic or have a mild dermatitis, often with dry, white scales on the dorsum of the back. Affected humans may develop a more prominent dermatitis, with grouped erythematous pruritic papules; occasionally, apical vesicles, bullae or urticarial wheals can be noted. The rash is commonly found in areas that have been in direct contact with the source animal, such as the chest, abdomen and upper extremities. Systemic hypersensitivity to *Cheyletiella blakei* has been reported, with associated peripheral blood eosinophilia and joint pain.

How do you treat for Cheyletiella?

Currently there are no products licensed for the treatment of cheyletiellosis in either cats or dogs. Spray, shampoo or spot-on formulations containing pyrethrins or pyrethroids are effective for treatment of cheyletiellosis on dogs; pyrethroids should not be applied to cats. Fipronil spot-on or spray formulations have been used for treatment of cheyletiellosis in dogs and cats. Spot-on treatment solution containing 10% imidacloprid has been shown to be effective for the treatment of canine cheyletiellosis, whereas spot-on selamectin solution has provided efficacy for the treatment of feline cheyletiellosis. The bedding and grooming equipment of infested animals should be disinfected.

Demodex – the follicle mite

Why is Demodex important?

Demodex canis is a minute, specialized burrowing mite, with a cigar-shaped body measuring 100–300µm in length and four pairs of stout legs ending in small blunt claws (Fig. 5.5). The opisthosomal region (behind the legs) is at least one-half of the body length and has a transversely striated cuticle. *Demodex* mites are unusual in that they live in the hair follicles and sebaceous glands of a wide range of wild and domestic animals, including humans, but in veterinary practice they are most important as a cause of skin disease in dogs. Feline demodicosis (caused by *Demodex cati* or *Demodex gatoi*) is an uncommon parasitic disease, though disease incidence in the UK, Europe and North America is increasing. Most dogs naturally carry a small number of *D. canis* without displaying clinical infestation. Under certain conditions, however, the mites can cause demodicosis (red mange),

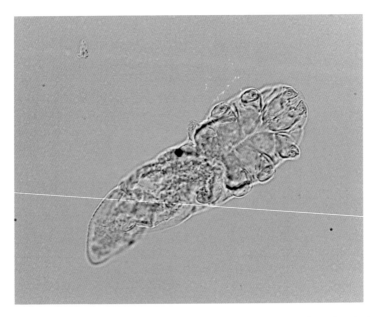

Fig. 5.5. Dog follicle mite, *Demodex canis*. *Demodex* spp. are tiny, cigar-shaped, eight-legged mites. They reside and feed in the hair follicle and oil glands of the skin.

regarded as one of the most important skin diseases in dogs. Demodicosis is more common in purebred dogs. These mites are unable to survive without their host and transmission is by direct contact. Female mites lay 20–24 eggs in the hair follicle, which develop via two six-legged larval stages followed by two nymphal stages. All stages of the life cycle may exist concurrently in one follicle and they feed head down. The life cycle is completed in 18–24 days. Transmission of *D. canis* from bitch to puppies occurs during the first 3 days of life through close physical contact while nursing. In their animal hosts, *Demodex* spp. usually cause little concern, living as a normal skin commensal. In susceptible dogs, however, for example those that are immunocompromised, it causes serious disease presentations.

How many types of demodectic mange are there?

Demodectic mange has been classified in various ways depending on the clinical manifestations. These categories include juvenile demodicosis, adult-onset demodicosis, localized demodicosis and generalized demodicosis. Juvenile demodicosis, which occurs in young dogs between 3 and 15 months of age, results in non-pruritic areas of focal alopecia on the head and forelimbs. The hind limbs and torso are rarely affected. The first lesions are frequently observed just above the eye, with small patches of depilation around the eye resulting in a 'spectacled' appearance. This form of the disease is self-limiting and recurrences are rare. Immunosuppressive therapy with glucocorticoids, however, may cause deterioration leading to generalized and pustular manifestations. Adult-onset demodicosis is often associated with concurrent staphylococcal pyoderma and is a pustular form of the disease. It can be localized or generalized with clinical signs including erythema, pustules, crusts and pruritus. The localized form is often confined in an area of one or two paws, whereas generalized conditions include six or more localized lesions on more than two affected limbs. The skin often becomes hyperpigmented in chronic cases. The generalized form commonly develops as a consequence of an underlying debilitating disease, such as hypothyroidism, hyperadrenocorticism, diabetes mellitus, prolonged immunosuppressive therapy, or neoplasia, or various infectious diseases, such as leishmaniosis, which reduce the host's immune defence mechanisms and are followed by a massive multiplication of mites.

Does Demodex from pets have any public health impact?

No. *Demodex* spp. are species specific. Humans have their own two species.

How do you diagnose demodicosis?

The diagnosis of demodicosis is based on the demonstration of large numbers of adult mites or significantly increased numbers in the immature stage as a proportion of adult mites. Deep skin scrapings taken from the edge of the lesions increase the chances of detecting the mites. Skin folds should be squeezed firmly to expel the mites from the depths of the hair follicles. Skin scrapings revealing low mite numbers should be considered normal hair fauna. Mites may also be detected by plucking hair samples for microscopic examination of the follicles.

How do you control demodicosis?

Localized demodicosis usually resolves spontaneously within 6–8 weeks, with or without the use of an acaricidal treatment. Treatment of generalized demodicosis is challenging and difficult and frequently requires extended and intensive therapeutic intervention. Amitraz, a formamidine derivative, is approved for the treatment of canine generalized demodicosis, applied as a dip at the rate of 250 ppm (0.025%) of active drug. About three to six applications that are 14 days apart may be necessary. Treatments should be preceded by a benzoyl peroxide shampoo to remove crusts and debris and to flush the follicles, allowing for better penetration of the acaricide. Treatment with amitraz washes carries a high success rate, though relapses after treatment are common. Some dogs will suffer skin reactions from treatment and its use is contraindicated in diabetic patients and Chihuahuas.

Protective clothing is required for the person who administers the product and washes should be applied in a well ventilated room. Human diabetics and asthma sufferers should not apply the product. Macrocyclic lactones have also been used successfully for treatment of generalized demodicosis. The spot-on formulation containing 10% imidacloprid + 2.5% moxidectin, applied topically at the recommended rate of 0.1 mg/kg, two to four times at 4-week intervals, provided clinical improvement, though weekly administration is also licensed and often required for clinical improvement to occur in more severe cases. Milbemycin oxime administered orally with dosages ranging from 0.5 to 2.2 mg/kg/day and treatment durations ranging from 9 to 26 weeks have been reported to be effective, but it is not licensed for this purpose in all European countries. Oral doses of ivermectin at 300 to 600 µg/kg/day with treatment duration extending 1 month beyond negative skin scrapings have also been effective but are not licensed in Europe or North America for this purpose.

The extra-label use of avermectins or milbemycins for the treatment of canine demodicosis should be approached with caution, especially for breeds with known sensitivity to these compounds. The isoxazolines are a recently developed class of insecticide for use against fleas and ticks and have also demonstrated excellent efficacy in the treatment of demodicosis. While currently an off-label use, it is likely that these products will become licensed for the treatment of demodicosis in the near future. While a dog is being treated for demodicosis, skin scrapings should be collected every 2–4 weeks, preferably from the same locations at each sampling site (at least one sample from the head and foreleg, respectively), undergoing microscopic examination for mites to monitor treatment progress. The total number of detectable mites, the ratio of live to dead mites and the ratio of adult *Demodex* mites to those in immature stages should be determined. These ratios can then be used to determine the success of the initial treatment. A quantitative reduction in the numbers of adult and immature mites or an abundance of dead mites is an indication of a successful healing process. A continued presence of numerous mites and a comparatively large number in the immature stages relative to adult mites may indicate further progression of the disease. Female dogs with generalized demodectic mange or a history of demodectic mange should be spayed, because the condition may worsen or relapse during oestrus or pregnancy and because of the inheritable predisposition of the disease.

Notoedres – a mange mite of cats

What is the importance of Notoedres cati?

Notoedres cati is similar in appearance to the scabies mite, *Sarcoptes scabiei*, and is the cause of face or head mange in cats, but other small animals such as pet rats and hedgehogs can also be affected. Females are about 230–300µm in size, whereas males are smaller. Notoedric mange manifests as alopecia and marked hyperkeratosis around the head and ears, with abundant epidermal scaling. Mites are transferred through direct contact and from infested females to kittens. Mites are identified by the round appearance, concentric striations on the dorsal cuticle and small stumpy legs. Very oddly, close examination will reveal that the anus is situated dorsally, i.e. on the back of the mite.

Otodectes – the ear mite

What is ear canker mite?

Otodectes cynotis (ear mite or ear canker mite) occurs worldwide in the external auditory canal of domestic dogs and cats; ferrets and other carnivores can also be affected. The mite is about 400 µm long, with a body flattened top to bottom and four pairs of long legs (Fig. 5.6). The epimeres (folds of cuticle) extending from the head region to the bases of legs 1 and 2 are joined. All developmental stages are found on the surface of the external ear canal, without being buried in the skin. The mite feeds on desquamated epithelial cells and aural exudates, but occasionally the mites pierce the skin to feed on blood, serum or lymph.

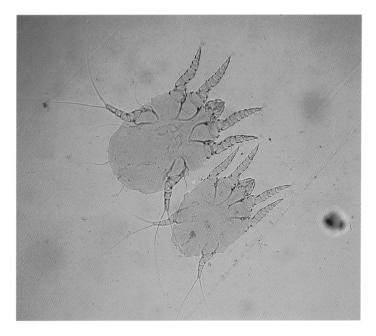

Fig. 5.6. The ear mite, *Otodectes cynotis*. This mite is about 0.4 mm long, with a body flattened top to bottom and four pairs of long legs. The male has a sucker on the end of each leg, while the female has suckers on only the first two pairs of legs. Living mites appear as small white organisms that can be seen moving within the ears or on swabs of deteritus removed from the ears.

What is the significance of ear mites?

This is a common mite infestation and the clinical importance of O. *cynotis* in pets is very high. O. *cynotis* is the cause of 50% of otitis externa cases in dogs and 85% of cases in cats. Mites are very annoying to cats: they cause severe irritation and thick, red crusts in the external ears. Eventually, infested ears droop and show a discharge. If the infestation is untreated, infection may spread from the outer to the inner ear, with possible serious bacterial involvement. The tympanic membrane may be perforated and otitis media and nervous signs (e.g. convulsions) can develop.

How do you control O. cynotis?

The ear canal of infested animals should be flushed and cleansed with a mild ceruminolytic agent. Traditional treatments have included using preparations of acaricides or mineral oil instilled directly into the ear canal. Frequent reapplications may be required. An otic suspension containing 0.01% ivermectin controls adult mites and also prevents the hatching of larvae from eggs. Systemic products providing extended residual activity are highly efficacious and convenient to apply. Topically applied imidaclo-prid + moxidectin solution is efficacious for treatment of otodectic mange in cats and topically applied selamectin solution is efficacious for the treat-ment of otodectic mange in cats and dogs. When a case of otoacariasis is confirmed, all dogs and cats in the household having direct contact should be treated. In addition, grooming equipment and bedding should be disin-fected, because mites are able to survive for a period of time off the host.

Sarcoptes scabiei – the itch mite

What is the life cycle and biology of S. scabiei?

S. scabiei, a burrowing itch mite, is the cause of sarcoptic mange or sca-bies and is able to infest a range of mammals. For small animal veterinary practices, it is sarcoptic mange in dogs that is of greatest concern. These mites have different degrees of host adaptation. Each subpopulation may be highly adapted to a particular host, so some strains may not easily infest a different species. Only one true species is recognized, but the mite often has 'var.' after the species name, which is an abbreviation for 'variety'. Hence, the mite found on dogs is often referred to as *S. scabiei* var. *canis*. Sarcoptic mange is rare in cats.

Adult female mites are 300–600 × 250–400 µm, whereas males measure 200–240 × 140–170 µm. These mites are unmistakeable in skin scrapings, being round, with the stumpy legs barely projecting beyond the body margins; the head is round but the main identification criteria are the scales and pegs or spines on the dorsal surface of the mite, which no other mange mite possesses (Fig. 5.7).

The life cycle of *S. scabiei* var. *canis* takes place exclusively on the dog, passing from egg to larva and through two nymphal stages in 2–3 weeks. After mating on the skin surface, the females burrow into the epidermis, making tunnels up to 1 cm long that are parallel to the surface. After a mat-uration phase of 4–5 days, the females deposit one to three oval eggs daily into these tunnels for about 2 months. The six-legged larvae hatch 3–4 days after oviposition and most of them crawl from the burrows to the skin sur-face, though some remain in the tunnels, where they continue to develop. The larvae moult first to protonymphs, then to tritonymphs and then to adults. They feed on damaged skin and tissue fluids. After mating, the newly developed males die, whereas the adult females look for a suitable site on the host for burrowing and subsequently depositing their eggs. The total egg-to-adult life cycle typically requires 17–21 days but may be as short as 14 days. Mites may survive off the host 2-3 weeks in sleeping areas and on grooming equipment, which should also be considered as potential sources of contamination.

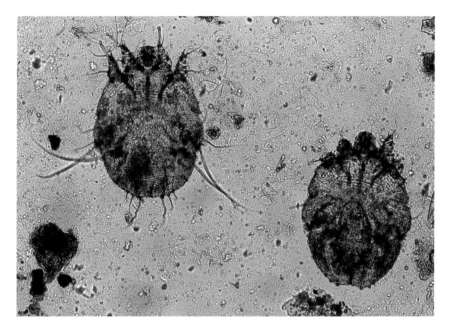

Fig. 5.7. The burrowing itch mite, *Sarcoptes scabiei*. Adult female *Sarcoptes* have triangular spines on the dorsal surface of the body.

What is the clinical presentation of sarcoptic mange?

Sarcoptic mange often begins on relatively hairless areas of skin on the head, with frequent distribution to the lower abdomen, chest and legs. The ears are almost always affected, particularly the inside of the pinna, as is the lateral aspect of the elbow. Lesions consist of follicular papules, yellow crusts of dried serum and excoriations from scratching due to intense pruritus. Secondary bacterial infections are frequent complications. The lesions usually spread rapidly, sometimes covering the entire body. The affected sites also display alopecia caused by self-inflicted trauma. Chronic cases result in thickening of the skin with hyperkeratosis, wrinkling and hyperpigmentation. In the most seriously affected skin areas, histopathological examination indicates severe chronic inflammation of the epidermis, with variable hyperkeratosis and parakeratosis. Despite obvious clinical lesions and intense pruritus, a diagnosis is often difficult. Dogs infested with these mites frequently display a 'pinnal–pedal' scratch reflex.

How are the mites detected?

Direct parasite detection should be performed with microscopic examination of skin scrapings taken from the edges of the lesions adjacent to intact tissue, i.e. not from open wounds or chronically inflamed excoriations. The preferred areas for obtaining skin scrapings are those covered with clearly visible raised yellowish crusts and papules. The accuracy of this diagnostic procedure depends on the number of examined skin scrapings and it is advisable to take at least ten scrapings per dog, though mites may not be found in approximately 50% of cases and diagnosis can be based on clinical manifestations and response to treatment. Unlike *Demodex* spp., the presence of a single mite is significant. An ELISA that detects *Sarcoptes* is also available.

Can other parasites cause skin thickening (hyperplasia)?

A hyperplastic response of the epidermis to arthropod infestation is a relatively common feature in a variety of mite, louse and flea infestations. Surprisingly, this same hyperplastic epidermal response may be elicited by parasites of a completely different phylum. For example, the nematode free-living parasite *Pelodera strongyloides* produces a nearly identical hyperplastic skin response when it opportunistically invades hair follicles in dogs, cattle, horses or humans. Generally, this skin invasion occurs when the host is lying in damp or filthy bedding and the skin is moist for prolonged periods of time. Initially a neutrophilic folliculitis develops, but then as the host self-traumatizes its skin, the same proliferative hyperkeratotic lesions as seen in sarcoptic mange will be apparent. Lesions develop as lichenified skin, with scaling, crusting and alopecia. Recently, a case of dual infection with both *Sarcoptes* and *Pelodera* in a wild black bear was reported, and the overall gross dermal lesions were indistinguishable from *Sarcoptes* alone. The skin appears to have a limited repertoire of patterns of inflammatory response, and self-trauma due to pruritis is a common manifestation of many ectoparasitic conditions.

How do you control this mite and treat the condition?

The coat should be clipped and crusty lesions and scale should be removed with an antiseborrheic shampoo. Traditional treatments have included the use of an acaricidal dip, such as lime sulphur, repeated weekly. Fipronil (0.25%) spray treatment (Frontline Spray, Merial) has been used successfully as an adjunct in treating sarcoptic mange alongside macrocyclic lactones. The preferred method of treatment includes the use of systemic macrocyclic lactones. A number of macrocyclic lactones have been demonstrated to be efficacious against sarcoptic mange, including monthly administration of selamectin or moxidectin (two to three treatments, 30 days apart, licensed in Europe and North America) and milbemycin (weekly treatment for 2 weeks, licensed in some European countries but not the UK). The isoxazolines have also been shown to be highly efficacious with one (sarolaner) being licensed and others likely to follow. All dogs having contact with infested dogs should be treated. Because mites are able to survive off the host, potential sources of contamination should be disinfected, including bedding, brushes and combs.

Trombicula

What is the Trombicula *spp. mite ('chiggers', 'Harvest mite' or 'Berry bug')?*

Cats and dogs are frequently infested on a seasonal basis with mites of the family Trombiculidae, more commonly known as 'chiggers' or 'harvest mites' (Fig. 5.8). Trombiculosis is highly unusual in that it is the larvae that cause the problem as they feed; the adults and nymphs are free-living predators of soft-bodied insects. The six-legged larvae are orange-red or yellow and measure 200–300 µm and are strongly seasonal in activity, generally encountered in late summer or autumn. At these times of year the larvae hatch from eggs on the ground, climb on vegetation and wait for passing hosts, in a similar way to some tick species. They are likely to be found on the ears, eyes, nose or other areas of thin skin, including the abdomen and regions between the toes. They usually occur in large clusters, easily spotted (although small) because they are orange. The larvae pierce the superficial epidermal layers with bladelike chelicerae to inject salivary gland enzymes into the skin. They then feed on liquefied tissues, body secretions and blood. After feeding, the engorged larvae drop to the ground to continue their development. Although only on the animal for a day or two, infestations often

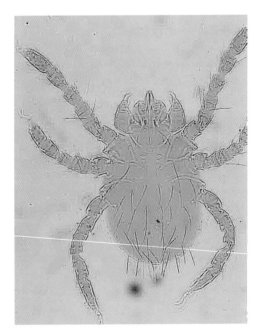

Fig. 5.8. Harvest mite, *Trombicula (Neotrombicula) autumnalis*. The six-legged chigger larva is 200–400 µm in diameter. The body is rounded and covered with tiny hairs, giving this mite a velvet-like appearance.

cause intense pruritus, erythema, excoriations and alopecia. Different responses to the infestations may be due to individual hypersensitivity reactions to the mites.

How do you prevent infestations of Trombicula spp?

This is rather difficult. Infested animals generally have a history of roaming through woods or fields in late summer. Topically applied fipronil and selamectin have been used successfully to treat trombiculosis in cats and dogs, and topical pyrethroid + pyriproxyfen formulations have been used to control these mite infestations on dogs. Traditional acaricide and insecticide formulations, including dips, sprays, powders and shampoos, have been used to treat and control these infestations.

Tick Infestations

What are ticks?

Like mites, ticks are acarines, not insects, having eight legs in the adult stage (insects, like lice and fleas, have six). Ticks are obligate blood-suckers and important vectors of diseases. There are two tick families of veterinary importance: the Argasidae (soft ticks) and Ixodidae (hard ticks). In Europe and North America, the most important tick species affecting dogs and cats (and also biting people) belong to the Ixodidae. Hard ticks are characterized by a dorsal shield (scutum) and a 'false' head (the basis capituli), which is actually the head fused with the thorax and which bears the palps. Palps are sensory in function and flank a toothed probe – the skin attachment structure, the hypostome. Some species are colourful and have eye spots on the scutum and indentations on the posterior margin, like the crust of a pie, called festoons. All these features can be used to aid identification, which is clinically important since certain notorious tick species are known vectors of serious pathogens and it is desirable to identify them, which can aid disease prognosis and help in surveillance.

How do ticks feed?

In order to feed, a tick locates a passing host by waving its front legs, a behaviour called 'questing'. The legs bear sensory organs called Haller's organs and can detect carbon dioxide and host kairomones. Ticks pierce the skin with their chelicerae and insert the hypostome. A secretory substance holds the hypostome in place and copious amounts of saliva are injected into the host. In addition to water, the saliva contains anticoagulant and immunomodulatory substances. The host may develop a localized reaction to the tick bite and there may be subsequent bacterial infection of the lesion. It should be noted that if a tick is forcibly removed the mouthparts may remain embedded and this may result in a foreign body reaction. Infestation with larvae or nymphs may go unnoticed, as these immature tick stages are small. Adult ticks, particularly engorging females, are most readily seen and may be of concern to owners. Understanding how ticks feed is important in understanding disease transmission.

What is the biology and significance of Ixodes ricinus *and other species in the UK?*

A number of tick species regularly attach to dogs and cats in the UK and countries of northern Europe but the most common is *Ixodes ricinus*, the sheep tick (Fig. 5.9a). *I. ricinus* is reddish brown, approx 4 mm in size when unfed, and pasture, woodland and scrub are all habitats for this species. Ticks that commonly occur in temperate climates all have a three-host life cycle: the larvae (Fig. 5.9b) feed on a host, drops off and moult to the nymph; the nymph feeds on another host and drop off to moult to an adult. All three stages attach to a different host at each feed. The immature stages feed on small mammals for 2–4 days but adults attach to larger hosts such as roe deer, which are increasing across Europe. Having mated while on the host, adult females feed for up to 10 days (usually 5–7 days); the large fed female tick then detaches and lays several thousand eggs in the environment before dying. The duration of the life cycle is highly dependent on environmental conditions, *I. ricinus* taking 3 years in the UK and Ireland to complete its life cycle (each stage feeds once per year) whilst taking only a year in Mediterranean countries. Cats and dogs become infested when they enter tick habitats and are then at risk of tick-borne diseases (TBDs). Increasing tick populations and TBDs are an emerging problem in the UK and Europe due to factors such as climate change, increase in woodland plantation, set-aside areas and increases in deer populations (an excellent feeding/maintenance host). *Dermacenor reticulatus* is another important species found in the UK and Europe and it also transmits *Babesia canis*, recently shown to be endemic in Essex, UK.

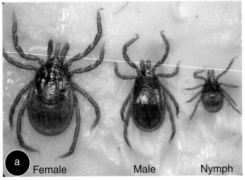 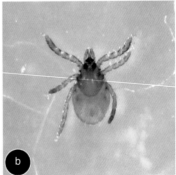

a Female   Male   Nymph   b

Fig. 5.9. (**a**) *Ixodes ricinus* adult versus nymph. (**b**) *Ixodes ricinus* larva.

What is tick-borne encephalitis (TBE)?

European TBE is transmitted by *I. ricinus* and *I. persulcatus* ticks present in forest and mountainous areas in western and central Europe. TBE is endemic in Austria, Belarus, Croatia, the Czech Republic, Estonia, Germany, Hungary, Latvia, Lithuania, Poland, western Russia, Slovakia, Slovenia, Switzerland and Ukraine. TBE does not occur in the UK but very occasionally (less than one per year) cases may be imported by UK travellers who have been to endemic areas. The majority of infected individuals do not have any symptoms, with the ratio of asymptomatic to symptomatic infection approximately 250:1. Most people with symptoms recover. However, up to one-third can suffer long-term complications due to the encephalitis. Treatment of those infected with TBE is supportive only. There is an effective vaccine available.

What is the significance and life cycle of brown dog tick, Rhipicephalus sanguineus, in Europe?

This species is a rarity in the UK but common in southern Europe and the USA. Infestations do arise from time to time in the UK, however, usually as a result of imported dogs. This tick is very different from *I. ricinus*, being adapted to living indoors, and may be found on dogs living in urban and rural environments. All stages feed mainly on dogs, or occasionally other hosts. It is a three-host species like *I. ricinus*. The fully fed females drop off at night and after a period of time will deposit thousands of eggs in crevices, cracks in dog kennels and under floor boards. Huge numbers of ticks can infest a single dog but most ticks are in the environment. The number of generations per year varies from region to region across Europe. *Rhipicephalus sanguineus* (Fig. 5.10) occasionally establishes in UK homes following dog travel abroad. Numbers increase quickly in warm rooms (e.g. kitchens) with untreated dogs. Global warming might prompt the establishment of populations in previously (largely) free areas, such as southern UK where temperatures just support the life cycle. The species is of great importance in southern Europe and indeed worldwide, as vector of pathogens such as *Babesia canis* and *Ehrlichia canis*.

What are the important tick species affecting dogs and cats in North America?

The tick species that most commonly infest dogs and cats in North America are *Amblyomma americanum* (Lone Star tick), *Amblyomma maculatum* (Gulf Coast tick), *Dermacentor occidentalis* (Pacific Coast tick), *Dermacentor variabilis* (American dog tick), *Dermacentor andersoni* (Rocky Mountain wood tick), *Ixodes pacificus* (western black-legged tick), *Ixodes scapularis* (black-legged tick), *Otobius megnini* (a soft tick, the spinose ear tick) and *Rhipicephalus sanguineus* (brown dog tick).

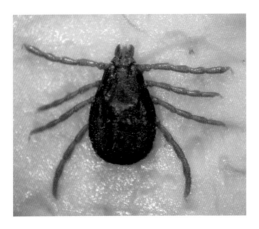

Fig. 5.10. Dorsal view of *Rhipicephalus sanguineus*. Also known as the brown dog tick or kennel tick. It is generally found in sheltered areas where climatic conditions remain relatively constant. Large concentrations of populations are found mainly in warm and moist environments.

How important is Amblyomma *in North America and what are the associated pathogens?*

A. americanum (Lone Star tick) is named for the characteristic and easily recognizable single white spot that occurs on the dorsal shield of the female. *A. americanum* has long palps, a long hypostome, eye spots and festoons. This tick occurs most commonly in woodland habitats with dense underbrush. Substantial reforestation over the past century, in urban and rural habitats, has provided increased areas of habitat for white-tailed deer and for survival and expansion of *A. americanum*. The white-tailed deer is considered a preferred host for *A. americanum* and all life stages will feed on it. Many other animals can be parasitized by this aggressive tick and immature stages can be found on various ground-dwelling birds and numerous mammals such as red fox, rabbits, squirrels, raccoons, dogs, cats, coyotes, deer and humans. Because all life stages can parasitize dogs and cats, *A. americanum* could be encountered on pets 8–9 months out of the year. Once hosts are acquired, larvae and nymphs engorge over a period of 3–9 days; adults typically engorge within 9 days, but may take up to 2 weeks to do so. As with most ticks, peak seasonal activity can vary widely by geographical region. Similar to other ixodid ticks, unfed adults may survive for prolonged periods (> 400 days) if hosts are not available. In temperate climates, the life cycle often takes 2 years to complete, whereas in warmer coastal climates it can be completed within 1 year.

A. americanum is considered a major vector of animal and human pathogens, including *Ehrlichia chaffeensis* (causing human monocytic ehrlichiosis) and *Ehrlichia ewingii*. The Lone Star tick can also transmit *Borrelia lonestari* and has been implicated in the transmission of *Francisella tularensis* (causing tularaemia). The Lone Star tick has also recently been demonstrated to be a competent vector of *Cytauxzoon felis*, the highly pathogenic and usually fatal protozoan parasite of cats. Another *Amblyomma* species, *A. maculatum*, transmits *Hepatozoon americanum*, the aetiological agent of American canine hepatozoonosis. The transmission of this disease is unique, in that dogs must ingest the tick to become infected. *A. maculatum* has also been documented to cause tick paralysis.

What is the life cycle and importance of Dermacentor in North America?

Dermacentor variabilis is an ornate (i.e. has a patterned scutum) ixodid tick. The scutum, which covers the entire dorsal surface of the male and the anterior one-third of the unengorged female, is covered with metallic grey-white markings. It also has festoons on the posterior abdomen, eyespots and short palpi. *Dermacentor* spp. are one of the most widespread and common ticks infesting dogs and cats in North America. They commonly occurs in grassy meadows, young forests and along roadways and trails. Common hosts for adult *D. variabilis* include cats, dogs, cattle, horses and other large mammals, including humans. Fully engorged *D. variabilis* females drop from their hosts within 4–10 days and deposit 4000–6500 eggs. The life cycle can be completed in 3 months in the southern USA but it may take up to 2 years in more northern climates. These ticks may carry a number of diseases that are readily transmitted when an infected tick feeds on a dog. These include Lyme disease, ehrlichiosis, anaplasmosis, Rocky Mountain spotted fever (RMSF) and babesiosis.

Should the dog's owner be concerned if bitten?

The dog is the preferred host of the adult *D. variabilis*, though this tick species feeds on many large mammals, including humans. This tick species is known to transmit RMSF and tularaemia to humans. It may also induce tick paralysis by elaboration of a neurotoxin that induces rapidly progressive flaccid quadriparesis.

What are the important Ixodes species in North America?

Ixodes scapularis, the black-legged tick (deer tick or Lyme disease tick), is an inornate tick without eyes or festoons. *I. scapularis* is widely distributed in at least 35 states in the eastern and central USA. It is also located in central and eastern Canada. Similar to *A. americanum*, the distribution of *I. scapularis* correlates with the distribution and abundance of white-tailed deer. Exclusion of deer dramatically decreases *I. scapularis* populations. The white-footed mouse (*Peromyscus leucopus*) is of particular importance in the tick's life cycle and disease transmission, because it serves as a host for larval *I. scapularis* and it is a major reservoir of *Borrelia burgdorferi*. *I. scapularis* is the vector of *B. burgdorferi* (causing Lyme disease) in the central, upper mid-western, and north-eastern USA; it is also the vector of *Anaplasma phagocytophilum* (causing human granulocytic ehrlichiosis) and *Babesia microti* (causing human babesiosis). *I. scapularis* may also cause tick paralysis. The western black-legged tick, *I. pacificus*, is morphologically similar to *I. scapularis*. It is the vector for *B. burgdorferi* and *A. phagocytophilum* in the western USA. *I. pacificus* ticks are distributed from Mexico to British Columbia, with localized populations in Utah and Arizona.

Is Rhipicephalus sanguineus *important in America?*

Yes, indeed worldwide. *R. sanguineus* (brown dog tick) is reddish brown and inornate, and has a hexagonally shaped basis capituli (false head). Eyes and festoons are present. These features distinguish it from *Ixodes* spp. *R. sanguineus* is the only tick that infests human dwellings and kennels in North America. It persists in temperate regions by inhabiting kennels and homes. The life cycle may be completed in as little as 63–91 days. This results in a rapid increase in tick populations and it can make infestations of homes or kennels extremely difficult to eradicate. *R. sanguineus* is the vector of *Ehrlichia canis* (causing canine monocytic ehrlichiosis) and *Babesia canis* (causing canine babesiosis). Also, it may transmit *Anaplasma* (formerly *Ehrlichia*) *platys* and *Babesia gibsoni*. Recently, in the south-western USA, this tick was identified as a vector for *R. rickettsii*, the causative agent of RMSF.

What environmental control strategies can be implemented for R. sanguineus *infestations?*

Successful strategies for brown dog tick control include appropriate use of environmental acaricides (i.e. synthetic pyrethroids) behind, under and around cages and in cracks and crevices in floors, walls and ceilings. Including the ceilings is particularly important, because brown dog ticks are inclined to climb upwards in indoor environments. Application of environmental tick control products should be performed by professional pest control specialists. It is also prudent to limit access to crawl spaces under homes, decks and outbuildings, to discourage visits by wildlife. Product properties or issues to be considered when designing regimens for successful tick control include numbers and species of ticks in the pet's environment, expected level of exposure to ticks, prevalence and spectrum of tick-borne diseases and severity of reactions to tick bites. Several published studies suggest that available tick control products can aid in the prevention of transmission of vector-borne diseases.

How did ticks become efficient disease vectors?

Ticks are notorious vectors of numerous infectious (bacterial, protozoal and viral) diseases in animals and humans. Many of the TBDs can cause significant economic consequences and are challenging to control. The important role of ticks in disease transmission is reinforced by the fact that ticks have a worldwide distribution, can adapt to diverse ecological niches and feed for extended periods of time and on a variety of vertebrate animals as they develop from juveniles to adults. Ticks' salivary glands play a major role not only in pathogen transmission and establishment, but also in the secretion of bioactive products of various critical functions, such as anti-haemostatic, anti-inflammatory and immunosuppressive. Ticks have a long, slow life cycle that takes several years in temperate climates. Because of this longevity, ticks can carry infectious organisms acquired from a huge range of wildlife hosts, over prolonged periods of time, thus not only acting as vectors but also serving as reservoir hosts for the pathogens they transmit. Some pathogens, like *Babesia* spp., persist in tick populations by passing from the adult tick into the eggs (transovarial transmission), an important epidemiological concept. Ticks can also benefit from the pathogens they carry. For instance, the presence of the bacterium *Anaplasma phagocytophilum* in some tick species increases the ability of ticks to survive in the cold temperatures by up-regulating an antifreeze-like glycoprotein. The increased survival of infected ticks allows the vectored pathogen to carry on in the environment.

What is borreliosis?

Lyme borreliosis is the most common tick-borne disease in Europe. A corkscrew-shaped gram-negative spirochete bacterium known as *Borrelia burgdorferi* is the pathogen causing this disease in animals and humans. Numerous clinical forms have been associated with Lyme disease in dogs. This multi-systemic disease causes fever, lameness, stiff joints, arthritis, fatigue, renal failure, heart disorders, meningitis and other neurological signs. Once the host contracts Lyme's disease, urgent treatment with antibiotics is required. Doxycycline or amoxicillin is the drug of choice, with doxycycline preferred in patients with evidence of renal disease as it is excreted almost entirely in the faeces. It is also reported to reduce joint inflammation in some cases. However, doxycycline should not be used in very young puppies because it can cause teeth staining. Other drugs, such as amoxicillin, ceftriaxone and high-dose penicillin, have been found to eradicate the disease and cure *Borrelia* infection in mice models. Non-steroidal anti-inflammatory drugs may also be used for symptomatic treatment. The current canine vaccine consists of killed *B. burgdorferi* in adjuvant.

What is Hepatozoon?

Hepatozoon canis can infect and cause disease in dogs worldwide. While all canine infections were attributed initially to *H. canis*, in 1997 a novel species, *H. americanum*, was identified in dogs in the southern USA. Contrary to *H. canis* infection, *H. americanum* typically results in a severe debilitating course of illness which, in the absence of treatment, is usually fatal.

What is Crimean Congo haemorrhagic fever (CCHF)?

CCHF is a viral infection transmitted by *Hyalomma* ticks and may arrive one day in the UK, carried by migrating birds and possibly establishing with climate change. It occurs in Eastern Europe and the Mediterranean. European outbreaks have also been reported in Albania, Greece, Kazakhstan, Kosovo and Turkey. CCHF is rare in travellers. However, in 1997, CCHF was reported in a UK traveller who had been to Zimbabwe. Symptoms are often mild, starting 1–3 days after a tick bite. Symptoms include fever, dizziness, headache, myalgia and photophobia. This can progress to haemorrhagic manifestations and death. The case fatality rate is between 20% and 35%. Treatment is supportive and there is no vaccine currently available.

What is tick paralysis?

Tick paralysis is not an infectious disease but is worth briefly considering, because ticks cause it and it affects dogs and cats, livestock and, in some cases, humans. This toxicosis is caused by neurotoxins produced by tick salivary glands and results in a rapidly ascending flaccid paralysis. To protect against *Ixodes holocyclus* tick-induced paralysis, research has been directed towards developing a vaccine using a recombinant inactive form of the toxin. However, other tick species, such as *R. sanguineus*, may also cause paralysis in dogs and thus require development of prevention measures.

Why don't dead ticks always fall off a host immediately?

Dead ticks do not always fall of the host immediately because they release a cement-like substance that can take up to 5 days to dissolve, even after the tick has died.

How do you remove ticks?

Ticks should be removed with either a simple 'twist and pull' action (if using a tick hook) or a straight gentle pull (if using fine-pointed tweezers). Ticks should not be crushed, squeezed, frozen or topically treated before removal as this will lead to regurgitation of stomach and salivary gland contents, increasing the risk of disease transmission. To avoid squeezing and crushing, blunt-ended tweezers or fingers should not be used to remove ticks.

How do you treat and prevent tick infestation?

Products include fipronil and imidacloprid (with permethrin) formulations, isoxazolines or synthetic pyrethroids, permethrin and deltamethrin (dogs only), and flumethrin incorporated into collars. Where *R. sanguineus* infestation has established in a house or kennels, environmental treatment with acaricide (preferably unrelated to the treatment used on the animals to avoid possible toxicity) may be necessary. Infestation levels should be monitored and treatment continued until there are no longer signs of tick infestation, bearing in mind that some infestations may be seasonal. The newer tick (and flea) control products, the isoxazolines, include afoxolaner with a claim of kill in 1–2 days, and with 1-month duration, as a chewable tablet, with the active ingredient entering the bloodstream, not the coat. In the same class is fluralaner, which will kill ticks within 12 h, protect for 3 months (2 months for *R. sanguineus*) and is administered orally as above. While highly efficacious and useful in reducing disease transmission, none of these products is 100% effective, making checking pets for ticks at least every 24 h and removing any found as described also important.

What should you do with the collected ticks?

It is always of value to identify ticks as this provides baseline data for surveillance purposes (https://www.gov.uk/guidance/tick-surveillance-scheme). The collected ticks should be preserved in glass vials containing 70% ethanol with a few drops of glycerine to maintain the natural colour and to prevent the hardening of the sample. Then, ticks should be identified using phenotypic identification keys for local tick species (e.g. http://www.bristoluniversitytickid.uk). Also, in the UK, animal owners and veterinary professionals can send ticks to Public Health England's Tick Recording Scheme or the Big Tick Project (http://www.bigtickproject.co.uk) for proper identification of the tick species.

Leishmaniosis

What is leishmaniosis?

Leishmaniosis is a Sandfly-borne disease of dogs caused by *Leishmania* spp. of the family Kinetoplastidae. Infection with *Leishmania* spp. can result in a spectrum of clinical diseases, dependent upon the infecting species. In Europe, three species have been reported: *L. infantum*, *L. tropica* and *L. donovani*. *L. infantum* is the only *Leishmania* species reported in both Old and New Worlds; it can potentially cause fatal leishmaniosis in dogs and visceral leishmaniasis (VL) and cutaneous leishmaniosis (CL) in humans. *L. tropica* and *L. donovani* occasionally cause CL and VL in humans.

How many Leishmania species can infect cats?

Five *Leishmania* species have been identified in cats: *L. mexicana*, *L. venezuelensis*, *L. braziliensis* and *L. amazonensis* in the New World, and *L. infantum* in both the New and Old Worlds. *L. infantum* is the only species isolated from cats in Europe.

What is the life cycle of Leishmania *parasites?*

The *Leishmania* life cycle involves a mammalian host and a vector stage. Phlebotomine sandflies (Fig. 5.11a) of the genus *Lutzomyia* in the Americas and *Phlebotomus* in other regions of endemicity in Europe serve as vectors for *Leishmania*. Sandflies are the only arthropods that are adapted to biological transmission of *Leishmania*. The sandfly injects infective promastigotes into a susceptible mammal during feeding. Promastigotes are then quickly phagocytized by resident phagocytes, transformed into tissue-stage (Fig. 5.11b) amastigotes, and divide through simple division in a parasitophorous vacuole. Sandflies become infected through feeding on a host either with an active skin lesion or with parasitaemia. Parasites convert to promastigotes within the sandfly midgut and reproduce to high numbers in 4–14 days. These promastigotes migrate to the salivary glands, transform into infectious metacyclic promastigotes and await the initiation of feeding.

Is there evidence of non-sandfly transmission in dogs?

Ticks and fleas have been evaluated as potential vectors of *Leishmania* but no evidence has been shown that they have a role in natural transmission of the protozoan. Direct dog-to-dog transmission has been implicated as being responsible for transmission of infection among foxhounds in the USA in the absence of apparent vectors; however, this has not been confirmed yet by experimental evidence. Transplacental transmission of infection in dogs is also possible and recently venereal transmission has also been reported in dogs. Transmission of infection by infected canine blood products has been documented and is of special concern in areas where blood donors could be carriers of infection. Nevertheless, non-sandfly modes of transmission probably play only a marginal role in the natural history and epidemiology of leishmaniosis.

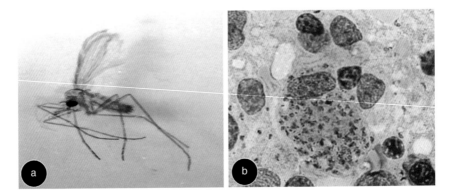

Fig. 5.11. (a) The phlebotomine sandfly, the insect vector of the protozoan parasites of genus *Leishmania*. (b) *Leishmania* amastigotes reside within infected macrophages of infected host.

How is leishmaniosis diagnosed?

The diagnosis of leishmaniosis takes into account the epidemiological context, clinical signs and results of laboratory tests. Information is collected about the animal's way of life (indoor/outdoor), history (particularly for the investigation of events that may have depressed its immune status, such as feline immuno-deficiency virus (FIV) infection, pregnancy or particular treatments such as cor-tico-therapy) and age. It is of first importance to know if the animal lives or has travelled in endemic areas. Leishmaniosis is characterized by various inconsistent and non-specific clinical signs. Furthermore, atypical forms of the disease can occur. Hence, the veterinary practitioner is most frequently led to request labora-tory tests to confirm its diagnosis. Blood, urine and tissue samples are collected for non-specific and specific laboratory tests. Infections such as feline immuno-deficiency virus or other blood infections (e.g. ehrlichiosis, hepatozoonosis, ba-besiosis) may also occur and should not be excluded before a definitive diagnosis.

What are the clinical signs in dogs?

Canine leishmaniosis is chronic in presentation with a variety of presenta-tions and periods of remission. Signs are due to immune complex deposition in various organs and include alopecia, hyperkeratosis, dermal ulcers, polyarthri-tis, ocular inclusion bodies, uveitis, hepatopathy, glomerulonephritis and neuro-logical signs associated with spinal and central nervous system granulomas. Peri-ocular alopecia (lunettes) are a classic sign and easily mistaken for atopy.

What are the predominant clinical signs in cats?

The most frequently described forms in feline leishmaniosis are cutaneous, consisting of ulcerative dermatitis, nodular dermatitis, alopecia and scaling. Animals are sometimes in poor condition with poly-lymphadenopathy, an-orexia and cachexia. Other forms of the disease such as ocular and visceral forms have been described and it is likely that new particular clinical ex-pressions will soon be described, given the recent interest in this disease in cats. Associated signs such as stomatitis and respiratory disease have also been observed. Subclinical infections may be usual in cat populations living in enzootic areas. For those animals, infection can develop into one of three patterns: progressing towards clinical disease; prolonged subclinical infec-tion; and elimination of the parasite.

What are the blood and urinary changes in dogs with leishmaniosis?

Non-specific laboratory tests (including complete blood count, serum biochem-ical panel, serum protein electrophoresis and urine) can lead to a suspicion of leishmaniosis and help to evaluate the physiological condition of the animal (particularly the renal function). Haematology generally shows regenerative or non-regenerative anaemia, lymphopenia, monocytosis and sometimes thrombocytopenia. Urinalysis can show moderate to severe proteinuria.

Which tools do you use to confirm diagnosis?

Specific diagnostic tools include microscopic examination of tissue samples, culture of the parasite, serology and PCR.

Cytopathology   The simplest method for the specific diagnosis of *Leishmania* is the demonstration of amastigotes in stained smears (Giemsa or May-Grünwald) from aspirates of hypertrophic lymph node or bone marrow. This technique offers a definitive diagnosis for a low cost and can be done quickly at veterinary clinics. However, it requires an experienced practitioner to be done properly.

Cultures   Parasites can be cultivated from bone marrow, lymph nodes or cutaneous biopsies in several media, but this technique is time consuming and lacks sensitivity. Therefore, it is rarely used for diagnosis, but is very useful for the isolation and identification of the parasite species.

Serology   The detection of anti-*Leishmania* antibodies (mainly IgG) can be performed using several techniques: agglutination tests, counter-immunoelectrophoresis, indirect immunofluorescence (IFAT), enzyme-linked immunosorbent assay (ELISA) and western blot. IFAT is widely used because it is easy to perform and offers good sensitivity and specificity. The test is genus specific, though cross-reactions may occur for individuals infected with parasites related to *Leishmania* (*Trypanosoma cruzi* or *T. rangeli*). All animals generally develop a humoral immune response and produce high antibody levels. However, a detectable level of antibodies in the blood may remain several months after the infection of the animal, especially for cutaneous forms of the disease. For cats particularly, the lack or low production of specific antibodies by infected animals could be related to the most common cutaneous clinical form of feline leishmaniosis rather than visceral.

Polymerase chain reaction (PCR)   PCR analysis can be used to detect the presence of the parasite *Leishmania* and to identify the genus or the species present. PCR on blood samples is not as sensitive for detection of *Leishmania* infection as samples from skin, lymph node and bone marrow. Conjunctival swabs have also demonstrated high sensitivity and are relatively non-invasive.

Which treatments are generally used?

Treatment has a variable prognosis depending on progression of disease, hepatic and renal function. Improvements in treatment success rates have made treatment a viable option and, as long as precautions are taken, zoonotic risk is minimal. No treatment is currently licensed for treatment of canine leishmaniosis in the UK. Treatment consists of allopurinol at 10–30 mg/kg in combination with meglumine antimonite (100mg/kg intravenous or subcutaneous) every 24 h for 3–6 weeks. All antimonial compounds are nephrotoxic and to a lesser extent hepatotoxic and so prognosis is worse in patients with concurrent hepatopathy and renal impairment. Renal and hepatic function should be closely monitored. Miltefosine (2 mg/kg every 24 h for 4 weeks) may be used instead of injectable treatments in combination with allopurinol and has the advantage in renal compromised patients of being metabolized solely by the liver. However, gastrointestinal side effects from its use are common. Treatment with allopurinol alone may be required for up to 6 months after resolution of clinical signs to prevent relapse and some patients will need to remain on the drug indefinitely. Supportive treatment for hepatic and renal function may also be required.

Several other drugs have been evaluated in therapeutic trials with various efficacies, such as aminosidine, ketoconazole, pentamidine, fluoroquinolones and metronidazole. However, leishmaniosis in humans, dogs and cats should be treated with varying drugs in order to reduce the risk of parasite resistance. For this reason, treatment based on amphotericin B is only prescribed to human patients and currently forbidden to treat animals in order to limit the development of resistant strains. All those drugs are only partially effective and it is generally assumed that the success of any chemotherapeutic regimen is dependent on the potential immunological response of the host, particularly the cell-mediated immunity, which involves macrophages and particular cytokines, such as IFN-γ. Therapy is often followed by a clinical improvement and a decrease in anti-*Leishmania* antibody titres. Treatment in cats and dogs is usually not followed by a parasitological cure and relapse of the clinical disease can occur. Follow-up of the treatment can be done by either serology or PCR.

According to the clinical signs, supportive treatment for renal function, appetite and symptomatic treatment may also be required. The skin sores caused by cutaneous leishmaniosis can heal without any treatment but this could take months, if not years. The infection by *Leishmania* parasites can sometimes spread from skin to the nose and/or the mouth and develop into mucosal leishmaniosis in worst cases. Occasionally surgical intervention is required to get rid of the sores. Strict hygiene should always be advised around patients and barrier nursing should be set up for hospitalized cases. Care must also be taken with sharps, as transmission can occur via contaminated needles.

Does any potential prevention system exist?

Disease prevention is essential for dogs travelling to endemic countries (e.g. Albania, Croatia, Cyprus, France, Greece, Italy, Malta, Portugal and

Spain). The best way to protect animals against the disease is to prevent the vector's bite by avoiding outdoor activities at night (because of the crepuscular activity of the sandfly), which is not always possible in enzootic areas. Fine-mesh insecticide-impregnated bed nets help to prevent bites, as does sleeping at altitude. Recently, a vaccine for the prevention of canine leishmaniosis (*L. infantum*) has been produced and is licensed throughout Europe but it has not yet been tested in cat populations. The use in dogs of a licensed deltamethrin collar every 5 months or application of a permethrin spot-on preparation every 2 weeks has been demonstrated to provide high levels of protection. In cats, the use of a sustained release flumethrin collar has been demonstrated to afford some protection off-licence.

Self-Assessment Questions

Fleas

1. Which of the following statements relating to *Ctenocephalides felis* (the cat flea) is most accurate?

(a) This flea is resistant to insecticidal agents currently available and high flea numbers are due to the products no longer working as they used to

(b) Some cat fleas are resistant to insecticidal agents currently available but usually infestations are due to incorrect use of the products

(c) There is no reported clinically significant resistance to insecticides currently available and infestations are usually due to incorrect use of the products

(d) *C. felis* can only be found on cats and therefore dogs cannot be infested with the cat flea

2. Which of the following most accurately reflects the time it takes to rid a house of a flea infestation?

(a) The average infestation takes 90 days to clear from a house

(b) Fleas are killed within 24 h so an infestation will be cleared within 1–2 days

(c) As the flea life cycle takes approximately 3 weeks to complete, most infestations will be cleared within 3 weeks in a home

(d) Once a home is infested it is not possible to clear the indoor infestation

3. **Which of the following most accurately reflects the time it takes to rid a pet of fleas?**

(a) Flea products act as repellents so you should never expect to see fleas on a correctly treated pet

(b) Most products kill fleas within 24 h provided they are used correctly and at the correct treatment interval; however, pets may constantly carry fleas if they are in an infested environment because no product acts as an effective repellant

(c) It can take 90 days to kill fleas on the pet

(d) There is no need to treat pets in the winter months as fleas are only a problem in spring and summer

4. **What is the primary source of cat fleas for reinfestation?**

(a) Pupae in the indoor environment

(b) Pupae in the outdoor environment

(c) Other pets – adult fleas usually jump from one pet to another

(d) Pupae in the indoor and/or outdoor environment, as adult fleas rarely jump from one animal to another

5. **What is the best way to manage the environment in established cat flea infestations?**

(a) Treat all the pets and prevent them from entering the home

(b) Treat all pets and use an insect growth regulator (IGR) as part of an integrated flea control approach, and vacuum/wash bedding

(c) There is no need to treat the pet as long as the environment is treated with an IGR and insect adulticide

(d) Turn down the heating in the home and reduce humidity to quickly clear the home infestation

Lice

1. **Which of the following statements relating to *Trichodectes canis* is most accurate?**

(a) This louse is able to infest a number of different animals as well as dogs

(b) It is a biting/chewing

(c) It is able to survive away from dogs for long periods of time

(d) It is the only clinically significant louse of dogs

2. **Which of the following insecticides is useful in treating** *Trichodectes canis* **infestations?**

   (a) Moxidectin

   (b) Selamectin

   (c) Fipronil

   (d) All of the above

3. **Which of the following statements is most true for the control of cat and dog lice infestation?**

   (a) The environment must be treated to eliminate persistent life cycle stages

   (b) Treatment all year round is essential to prevent lice reinfestation

   (c) All in-contact pets of the same species should be treated when an infestation is identified

   (d) Owners may also become persistently infested with cat or dog lice

4. **What is the primary source of cat and dog lice for reinfestation?**

   (a) Lice in the indoor environment

   (b) Lice in the outdoor environment

   (c) Contact with wildlife reservoir hosts

   (d) Close contact with other infested pets

5. **Which of the following statements about dog lice is true?**

   (a) Both sucking and biting lice species may be present

   (b) Only biting lice are clinically significant

   (c) Only sucking lice are clinically significant

   (d) Dog lice may also infest cats and people

Mites

1. **Which of the following mites live in hair follicles?**

   (a) *Demodex* spp.

   (b) *Trombicula* spp.

   (c) *Otodectes cynotis*

   (d) *Sarcoptes scabiei*

2. **Which of the following is a burrowing mite?**

   (a) *Cheyletiella* spp.

   (b) *Trombicula* spp.

   (c) *Otodectes cynotis*

   (d) *Sarcoptes scabiei*

3. **What percentage of otitis externa cases in cats is due to ear mites?**

   (a) 65%

   (b) 75%

   (c) 85%

   (d) 95%

4. **Which of the following mites have a free living stage?**

   (a) *Demodex* spp.

   (b) *Trombicula* spp.

   (c) *Otodectes cynotis*

   (d) *Sarcoptes scabiei*

5. **How long can sarcoptic mange mites live for off the host?**

   (a) 1–2 days

   (b) 3–4 days

   (c) 5–7 days

   (d) 2–3 weeks

Ticks

1. **Which is the most common tick infesting cats and dogs in the UK?**

   (a) *Dermacentor reticulatus*

   (b) *Dermacentor variablis*

   (c) *Ixodes hexagonus*

   (d) *Ixodes ricinus*

2. **Which of the following ticks transmits *Ehrlichia chaffeensis*?**

   (a) *Amblyomma americanum*

   (b) *Dermacentor reticulatus*

   (c) *Dermacentor variablis*

   (d) *Rhipicephalus sanguineus*

3. **Which of the following is an effective treatment for Lyme disease?**

   (a) Fenbendazole

   (b) Doxycylcine

   (c) Levamisole

   (d) Allopurinol

   (e) Albendazole

4. **Which of the following organisms appear as piroplasms in stained blood films?**

   (a) *Babesia* spp.

   (b) *Borrelia* spp.

   (c) *Ehrlichia* spp.

   (d) *Hepatozoon* spp.

5. **Which of the following ticks transmits tick-borne encephalitis?**

   (a) *Dermacentor reticulatus*

   (b) *Dermacentor variablis*

   (c) *Ixodes hexagonus*

   (d) *Ixodes ricinus*

Leishmaniosis

1. **What is the vector of *Leishmania* spp.?**

   (a) Fleas

   (b) Mosquitoes

   (c) Sandflies

   (d) Ticks

2. **Which of the following is a treatment for leishmaniosis?**

   (a) Fenbendazole

   (b) Doxycycline

   (c) Milbemycin oxime

   (d) Miltefosine

3. **Which of the following treatments for leismaniosis is restricted for human use only?**

   (a) Fenbendazole

   (b) Amphotericin B

   (c) Milbemycin oxime

   (d) Miltefosine

4. **Which dog breed is resistant to *Leishmania*?**

   (a) Ibizan hound

   (b) German shepherd dog

   (c) Cocker spaniel

   (d) Boxer

5. **Which body organ is known to be impacted by treatment of leishmaniosis?**

   (a) Heart

   (b) Liver

   (c) Kidney

   (d) Spleen

6 Parasites of the Eye and Nervous System

Thelaziosis

What is thelaziosis?

Thelaziosis, also known as eye worm infection, is caused by nematodes of the genus *Thelazia*, which are transmitted by flies into the orbital cavities and surrounding tissues of many species of wild and domestic mammals. Out of 16 species of *Thelazia* described so far, *T. rhodesii* infects sheep; *T. skrjabini* infects cattle; *T. californiensis* and *T. callipaeda* infect carnivores, including dogs, cats, foxes and wolves, and also rabbits. The disease is mainly seen in summer and autumn when the vector flies are active. It has been suggested that more than one species of Diptera is involved in its transmission; for example, the facefly, *Musca autumnalis*, transmits the worm to cattle, and *Phortica variegata* (Drosophilidae family) is a proven vector of the nematode in dogs and wild carnivores.

How are eye worms transmitted?

Adult worms live in the eyes under the nictitating membrane. The females release first-stage larvae (L1). When other flies feed on lachrymal secretions, they pick up the L1s which then go through two moults inside the fly, eventually to the third-stage infective larvae (L3). When the fly feeds again, the L3 larvae are transferred to an animal and develop into adult worms.

What are the clinical features, pathology and diagnosis of eye worms?

Infection is often unapparent, but worms may cause lacrimation, mucopurulent discharge, epiphora, conjunctivitis, keratitis, corneal opacity and ulcers and photophobia. As a result, infected animals can lose their vision. Eye worm infection can be differentiated from infectious keratitis by observing the adult worm (white, approximately 1 cm) in the conjunctival sac or demonstrating first-stage larvae in eye washings. The site of development is usually diagnostic for *Thelazia* spp. but aberrant migrating worms such as ascarids, *Angiostrongylus vasorum* and *Dirofilaria repens* can also be found in the eye.

How do you treat infections?

Treatment of canine thelaziosis is currently based on the mechanical removal of nematodes directly from the eyes of affected animals, after medication by local anaesthetic, but this is an invasive option. Local instillation of anti-parasitic drugs and subcutaneous administration of ivermectin have been described and more recently ocular instillations of moxidectin have proved to be highly effective in the control of canine thelaziosis. Oral milbemycin oxime is also now licensed for the treatment of *Thelazia* in dogs.

Can people become infected?

Yes, but uncommonly. Some *Thelazia* species (*T. californiensis* and *T. callipaeda*) cause human thelaziosis resulting in conjunctivitis, pain and excessive lacrimation. Humans are believed to be an accidental host but cases of human infection are increasingly reported across Europe, most recently in the Baltic States.

Encephalitozoonosis

What is encephalitozoonosis?

Canine encephalitozoonosis is a protozoal infection caused by the obligate intracellular microsporidial parasite, *Encephalitozoon cuniculi*, and has occasionally been identified as a cause of neurological or renal disease in dogs, with fatal consequences in puppies. Infection during pregnancy can lead to fetal death and stillbirths. *E. cuniculi* is best known as a cause of granulomatous encephalitis and nephritis in rabbits and rodents but this is also the main clinical presentation in dogs and may be confused with canine distemper. There are at least three strains of *E. cuniculi*, with strain 1 being limited to lagomorphs and strains 2 and 3 potentially infecting humans and dogs. Dogs are thought to become infected from environmental contamination with cysts, primarily from the urine of reservoir hosts.

How do you diagnose encephalitozoonosis?

Parasite spores can be detected in faeces and/or urinary sediments from infected dogs. Other tests include *in vitro* culture of parasites from fresh brain and/or kidney tissues and serological detection of anti-parasite antibodies. Definitive identification of *Encephalitozoon* is achieved by ultra-structural examination, whereas species and strain identification are dependent on DNA analysis using PCR.

How do you treat this disease?

Treatment is primarily supportive treatment for renal disease and steroids to limit granulomatous inflammation and neurological signs. Specific neurological signs, such as seizuring, may require symptomatic treatment. No anthelminitc has been licensed for use against the parasite in dogs and there are no large studies on the efficacy of benzimadazoles in canine patients. Albendazole (a benzimidazole) is not approved for use in dogs but it might be an off-label treatment option as it has some efficacy in human patients. Similarly, fenbendazole may be useful but there are no data on doses or duration of treatment required to treat *E. cuniculi* infection in dogs.

Is encephalitozoonosis zoonotic?

Human infection, via ingestion or inhalation of infective *E. cuniculi* spores, has been reported, particularly in immunocompromised patients. It is currently thought that pigeons, rather than pet mammals, present the largest reservoir of infection for human patients. Good hand hygiene should be practised around patients with suspected *E. cuniculi* infection.

Neosporosis

What is neosporosis?

Neospora caninum is a protozoal parasite closely related to *Toxoplasma gondii* and is an important cause of abortion in dairy cattle. The definitive host for *N. caninum* is the dog, which sheds oocysts. Recognized intermediate host are cattle and horses.

What are the clinical signs of neosporosis in dogs?

Most cases of clinical neosporosis occur in puppies less than 6 months old, infected transplacentally. Disease can occur in older dogs but this tends to occur due to immune suppression or concurrent illness. Typical clinical signs include progressive hind limb paresis and ataxia but muscle atrophy, spinal pain, ocular abnormalities and dysphagia may also occur. In puppies, the ascending paralysis caused in neosporosis can often be fatal and carries a poor prognosis.

How do you diagnose clinical disease in dogs?

Oocysts in faeces are infrequently shed and very rarely detected, and even then may be confused with those of *Hammondia* spp. PCR can be carried out on cerebrospinal fluid or muscle biopsies to detect the tissue cysts (Fig. 6.1) and serology (IFAT or ELISA) is also a useful indicator in combination with clinical signs. Puppies usually seroconvert 2–3 weeks following infection with antibody levels usually being high in clinically affected dogs.

How do you treat and prevent neosporosis?

The prognosis in clinical cases is guarded and treatment outcomes are improved if treatment is started early. It is therefore preferable to start treatment if neosporosis is suspected rather than waiting for laboratory confirmation. Treatment with clindamycin (20 mg/kg twice daily for 30–60 days) has some efficacy. To prevent spread of infection, chronically infected bitches should be prevented from breeding and dogs should be fed meat that has been cooked, or meat that has been frozen at least to –18°C for 48 h. Farm dogs should be denied access to bovine aborted materials; and faecal contamination of water courses and cow feed by dogs should be prevented.

Toxoplasmosis

What is toxoplasmosis?

Toxoplasmosis is a disease caused by a single-celled parasite called *Toxoplasma gondii*. Toxoplasmosis is one of the most common parasitic

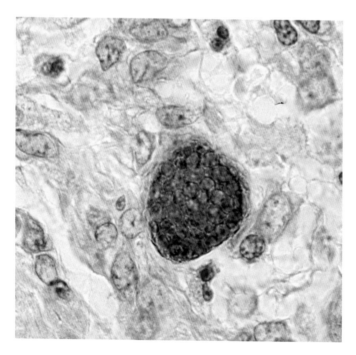

Fig. 6.1. Tissue cyst of *Neospora caninum*, the causative agent of neosporosis.

diseases and has been found in nearly all warm-blooded animals, including pets and humans. Despite the high prevalence of *T. gondii* infection, clinical disease caused by the parasite is relatively uncommon. The life cycle of *T. gondii* is complex and involves two types of host: definitive and intermediate. Cats, both wild and domestic, are the only definitive (final) hosts for *T. gondii*. When a cat ingests infected prey (or other infected raw meat), the parasite is released into the cat's digestive tract. The organisms then multiply in the wall of the small intestine and produce oocysts during what is known as the intra-intestinal infection cycle. These oocysts are then excreted in great numbers in the cat's faeces. Cats previously unexposed to *T. gondii* will usually begin shedding oocysts 3–10 days after ingestion of infected tissue and continue shedding for around 10–14 days, during which time many millions of oocysts may be produced in the environment. These oocysts (Fig. 6.2a) are very resistant and may survive for well over a year.

During the intra-intestinal infection cycle in the cat, some *T. gondii* organisms released from the ingested cysts penetrate more deeply into the wall of the intestine and multiply as tachyzoite forms (Fig. 6.2b). These forms then spread out from the intestine to other parts of the cat's body, starting the extra-intestinal infection cycle. Eventually, the cat's immune system restrains this stage of the organism, which then enters a dormant or 'resting' phase by forming cysts in muscles and brain (Fig. 6.2c). These cysts contain bradyzoites, which are slowly multiplying organisms. Other animals, including humans, are intermediate hosts of *T. gondii* and can become infected but do not produce oocysts (only felines do this). Oocysts passed in a cat's faeces are not immediately infectious to other animals but must first go through a process called sporulation, which takes 1–5 days, depending on environmental conditions. Once sporulated, however, oocysts are infectious to cats, people and other intermediate hosts. When intermediate hosts become infected through ingestion of sporulated oocysts,

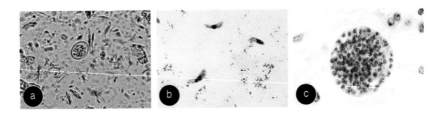

Fig. 6.2. (a) *Toxoplasma gondii* oocyst that is produced only through sexual reproduction in cats. *T. gondii* oocysts are shed in cat faeces and can remain viable in soil and water samples for months to years. (b) *T. gondii* tachyzoites. They are responsible for acute infection by rapidly multiplying inside neural and muscle tissue of infected hosts and when subjected to pressure from host immune system or treatment they transform into bradyzoites within tissue cysts. (c) The tissue cystic stage of *T. gondii* (agent of toxoplasmosis) showing a cyst wall enclosing numerous bradyzoites. (Courtesy of Dr J.P. Dubey, USDA, Beltsville, Maryland.)

infection results in formation of cysts in various tissues of the body and they remain in the intermediate host for life. Tissue cysts containing bradyzoites are infectious to cats, people and other intermediate hosts when the cyst-containing tissue is eaten.

How will toxoplasmosis affect a cat?

Most cats infected with *T. gondii* will not show any clinical signs but these do occasionally occur, particularly when the cat's immune response is not adequate to stop the spread of mobile tachyzoite forms. The disease is more likely to occur in cats with suppressed immune systems, including young kittens and cats with feline leukaemia virus (FELV) or feline immunodeficiency virus (FIV). The most common symptoms of toxoplasmosis include fever, loss of appetite and lethargy. Other symptoms may occur, depending on whether the infection is acute or chronic and where the parasite is found in the body. In the lungs, *T. gondii* infection can lead to pneumonia, which will cause respiratory distress of gradually increasing severity. Toxoplasmosis can also affect the eyes and central nervous system, producing inflammation of the retina or anterior ocular chamber, abnormal pupil size and responsiveness to light, blindness, incoordination, heightened sensitivity to touch, personality changes, circling, head pressing, twitching of the ears, difficulty in chewing and swallowing food, seizures and loss of control over urination and defecation.

How do you diagnose toxoplasmosis in cats?

Toxoplasmosis is usually diagnosed based on the history, signs of illness and the results of supportive laboratory tests. Measurement of IgG and IgM antibodies to *T. gondii* in the blood can help to diagnose toxoplasmosis. The presence of significant IgG antibodies to *T. gondii* in a healthy cat suggests that the cat has been previously infected and now is most likely immune and not excreting oocysts. The presence of significant IgM antibodies to *T. gondii*, however, suggests an active infection of the cat. The absence of *T. gondii* antibodies of both types in a healthy cat suggests that the cat is susceptible to infection and thus would shed oocysts for 1–2 weeks following infection. Sometimes the oocysts can be found in the faeces but this is not a reliable method of diagnosis, because they look similar to some other parasites. Also, cats shed the oocysts for only a short period of time and often are not shedding the oocysts when they are showing signs of disease. A definitive diagnosis requires histopathological examination of tissues or tissue impression smears for distinctive pathological changes and the presence of tachyzoites.

Can toxoplasmosis be treated?

Most cats that have toxoplasmosis can recover with treatment. Treatment usually involves clindamycin at 12.5–20 mg/kg twice daily. Other drugs that are used include pyrimethamine and sulfadiazine, which act together to inhibit *T. gondii* reproduction. Treatment must be started as soon as possible after diagnosis and continued for several days after signs have disappeared. In acute illness, treatment is sometimes started on the basis of a high antibody titre in the first test. If clinical improvement is not seen within 2–3 days, the diagnosis of toxoplasmosis should be questioned. No vaccine is as yet available to prevent either *T. gondii* infection or toxoplasmosis in cats, humans or other species.

Can you 'catch' toxoplasmosis from a cat?

Because cats only shed the organism for a few days in their entire life, the chance of human exposure from an individual cat is small. Owning a cat does not mean that its owner will be infected with the parasite. It is unlikely that a person would be exposed to the parasite by touching an infected cat, because cats usually do not carry the parasite on their fur, and it is also unlikely that a person could become infected through cat bites or scratches. In addition, cats kept indoors that do not hunt prey or are not fed raw meat are not likely to be infected with *T. gondii*. People are much more likely to become infected through their food than from handling cat faeces. Good hand hygiene, however, is important to minimize risk when cleaning litter trays and handling cat faeces, especially for pregnant women, immune-deficient individuals or those working in industries and careers that bring them into contact with large numbers of cats.

How are people infected with T. gondii?

Contact with oocyst-contaminated soil is probably the major means by which many different species – rodents, ground-feeding birds, sheep, goats, pigs and cattle, as well as humans living in developing countries – are exposed to *T. gondii*. In industrialized nations, most transmission to humans is probably due to eating raw or undercooked infected meat, particularly lamb and pork. People also become infected by eating unwashed fruit and vegetables. The organism can sometimes be present in some unpasteurized dairy products, such as goat's milk. *T. gondii* can also be transmitted directly from a pregnant woman to the unborn child when the mother becomes infected during pregnancy. There are two populations at high risk for infection with *T. gondii*: pregnant women and immune-deficient individuals.

Congenital infection is of greatest concern in humans, with about one-third to one-half of human infants born to mothers who have acquired *T. gondii* during that pregnancy being infected. The vast majority of women infected during pregnancy have no symptoms of the infection themselves.

The majority of infected infants will show no symptoms of toxoplasmosis at birth but many are likely to develop signs of infection later in life. Loss of vision, mental retardation, loss of hearing, and death in severe cases, are the symptoms of toxoplasmosis in congenitally infected children. In immune-deficient people such as those undergoing immunosuppressive therapy (e.g. for cancer or organ transplantation) or those with an immunosuppressive disease such as AIDS, enlargement of the lymph nodes, ocular and central nervous system disturbances, respiratory disease and heart disease are among the more characteristic symptoms. In these patients, especially those with AIDS, relapses of the disease are common and the mortality rate is high. In the past, immune-deficient people and pregnant women were traditionally advised to avoid cats but it is now not considered necessary as long as good hand hygiene is maintained.

How common is toxoplasmosis during pregnancy?

The risk of getting toxoplasmosis during pregnancy is very low. A 2010 study showed that, in non-immune women (those who have not had the infection before), about five per 1000 may get *T. gondii* infection, with a 10–100% risk of transmission to the baby. In the UK, about three in every 100,000 babies are born with congenital toxoplasmosis.

How do you prevent toxoplasmosis?

It is important to know measures that can be taken to help reduce the risk of developing a toxoplasmosis infection. These measures are particularly important for those who are pregnant or have a weakened immune system.

- Wear gloves when gardening, particularly when handling soil – wash hands thoroughly afterwards with soap and hot water.
- Avoid eating raw or undercooked meat, particularly lamb and pork, including any ready meals.
- Wash hands before and after handling food.
- Wash all kitchenware thoroughly after preparing raw meat.
- Always wash fruit and vegetables before eating them, including pre-prepared salads.
- Avoid drinking unpasteurized goat's milk or eating products made from it.
- Wear gloves when changing a cat's litter tray and wash hands thoroughly afterwards; if pregnant or with a weakened immune system, ask someone else to change the litter.
- Give cats dried or canned cat food rather than raw meat to ensure they do not eat infective meat.

- Cover children's sandpits to stop cats using them as a litter box.
- If pregnant, avoid coming into contact with sheep and newborn lambs during the lambing season, as there is a small risk that an infected sheep or lamb could pass the infection on at this time.

Self-Assessment Questions

1. *Thelazia* infection is associated with which part of the body?

(a) Eye

(b) Heart

(c) Kidney

(d) Skin

2. Which of the following anthelminitics is licensed to treat thelaziosis in dogs?

(a) Albendazole

(b) Fenbendazole

(c) Praziquantel

(d) Milbemycin oxime

3. *Neospora caninum* is closely related to which of the following protozoa?

(a) *Leishmania infantum*

(b) *Giardia* spp.

(c) *Toxoplasma gondii*

(d) *Isospora canis*

4. Which of the following has some efficacy in treating *N. caninum* infection?

(a) Clindamycin

(b) Fenbendazole

(c) Levamisole

(d) Praziquantel

5. *Toxoplasma gondii* infection is mainly associated with which part of the body?

(a) Brain

(b) Skin

(c) Eye

(d) Spleen

7 Parasites of the Urogenital System

Capillariasis

What are the Capillarid species in dogs and cats?

Capillarid worms that have a veterinary significance are *Capillaria aerophila = Eucoleus aerophilus* (lung), *C. hepatica* (liver) and *C. plica* (kidney). *Capillaria* spp. have a worldwide distribution.

What is C. plica *and what problems does it cause?*

C. plica is a parasite that resides in the urinary bladder, ureters or, rarely, in the kidney pelvis of various wild carnivores. Fox populations act as a major wildlife reservoir of infection. As a result, dogs living in areas with high densities of foxes, or frequenting environments visited by foxes, may be at greater risk of infection as the number of infected intermediate hosts subsequently increases. The life cycle of this parasite is indirect and involves an earthworm as intermediate host; transmission occurs following the ingestion of an infected earthworm containing first-stage larvae. After two moults and a short dwelling period in the intestine, third-stage larvae reach the bladder, where they moult to adults and embed themselves deep into bladder mucosa (occasionally ureters and kidney pelvis).

C. plica in dogs is of relatively minor clinical significance. However, haematuria, dysuria, or even renal failure associated with glomerular amyloidosis may develop with or without periodic signs of clinical cystitis or secondary bacterial cystitis. Urinary sediment examination is the only diagnostic tool that permits the identification of *C. plica* eggs (Fig. 7.1). Since the excretion of *C. plica* eggs varies considerably from day to day, the sensitivity of urinary sediment examination for diagnosing this infection can be low and hence a reliance on finding eggs when this condition is suspected (or when it is necessary

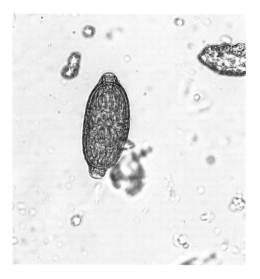

Fig. 7.1. Egg of *Capillaria plica*. The eggs are colourless with two bipolar plugs and rough surface ('netted' in appearance) and measure 65 μm × 25 μm.

to confirm treatment efficacy) must be in this context. More than one examination of urine sediment should be performed. Urinalysis may also reveal mild proteinuria, microscopic haematuria and the presence of an increased number of transitional epithelial cells. Success in treating *C. plica* infection has been reported using benzimidazoles. In dog shelters where *C. plica* is endemic several measures can be taken to avoid infection and reinfection from the environment, such as limiting contact of dogs with earthworms.

What other Capillaria spp. are of veterinary significance?

C. hepatica occurs in wild rats. It is not a lungworm; rather, adult worms reside in the liver. Specific diagnosis of *C. hepatica* infection is based on demonstrating adult worms and/or eggs in liver tissue at biopsy or necropsy. Other animals (and humans) have been infected with this species, usually by ingesting eggs released into soil from decaying rodents.

Dioctophymosis

What type of worm is Dioctophyma renale?

Dioctophyma renale is the largest known parasitic nematode in domestic animals and is known as the "giant kidney worm" of dogs. Adult females can measure up to 60 cm long and 12 mm wide, whereas males only reach 30 cm long and 6 mm wide. This parasite is unique in that it is found in the kidney, as its colloquial name implies, and it affects canines and mustelids. It occurs in temperate areas and subarctic areas, mainly northern USA and Canada.

How do adult D. renale *get into the kidneys?*

The life cycle of the worm is complex and includes intermediate, paratenic and definitive hosts. Eggs of *D. renale* are passed in the urine and ingested by the intermediate host, which are aquatic oligochaetes (mud-worms), where the nematode develops until the fourth larval stage. Oligochaetes are then eaten by paratenic hosts (fish or frogs), where the infective larvae are encysted in tissues of these animals without further development. Definitive hosts (fish-eating carnivores) are infected by ingestion of contaminated oligochaetes or paratenic hosts. In these animals, the larva penetrates the duodenal wall, enters the abdominal cavity and migrates to the kidney, where it remains until the adult stage. The adult worm is commonly found in the renal pelvis. In dogs, the right kidney is more affected than the left one, due to its anatomic proximity to the duodenum.

What kind of damage do you expect to see in the kidney of affected dogs?

The main lesion is the progressive destruction of the renal parenchyma, leaving only a thin capsule containing the worm and haemorrhagic exudates inside.

What signs does a dog with dioctophymosis infection exhibit?

Death has been associated with urine retention and uraemia due to chronic renal insufficiency. When one kidney is affected, the signs of renal failure may not be evident but haematuria can occur. If the parasite migrates to the peritoneal cavity, abdominal distension and peritonitis can be observed.

How do you diagnosis dioctophymosis?

The diagnosis is difficult due to the non-specificity of the clinical signs, especially in unilateral renal manifestation. Diagnosis can be achieved via detection of worm at necropsy; diagnostic imaging (radiography and ultrasound) may aid in localizing the presence of the parasite in the renal parenchyma. Urinalysis is conclusive, where the parasite eggs are seen in the animal's urine. However, eggs (80 μm, pitted shell and embryonated) will only appear in the urine sediment if a gravid parasite female is in the kidney causing the infection.

How do you manage a dog with dioctophymosis?

There is no known therapy for animals infected with *D. renale* but in cases of unilateral renal infection, nephrectomy of the affected kidney can be done. In some cases it is necessary to perform an exploratory laparotomy or nephrotomy to remove the parasites. Control includes limiting the contact of dogs with intermediate and transport hosts.

What are the public health implications of Dioctophyma renale?

D. renale cases have been described in humans.

Self-Assessment Questions

1. ***Dioctophyma renale* infection is associated with which part of the body?**

   (a) Eye

   (b) Heart

   (c) Kidney

   (d) Skin

2. **Which of the following anthelmintics is useful in treating *D. renale* infection?**

   (a) Fenbendazole

   (b) Praziquantel

   (c) Milbemycin oxime

   (d) None are known to be effective

3. **How is *D. renale* infection acquired by dogs?**

   (a) Mosquito bites

   (b) Drinking water

   (c) Faecal–oral route

   (d) Consumption of mud-worms, amphibians or fish

4. **Which of the following is known as the 'bladder worm'?**

   (a) *Capillaria plica*

   (b) *Toxocara canis*

   (c) *Dioctophyma renale*

   (d) *Echinococcus multilocularis*

5. **Which of the following act as intermediate host in the life cycle of *Capillaria plica*?**

    (a) Brown ants

    (b) Earthworms

    (c) Slugs

    (d) Aquatic snails

8 Key Skills for the Veterinary Nurse in Diagnostic Parasitology

This chapter will firstly explain some simple diagnostic tests, which may be carried out for parasites in practice and include faecal analysis, staining blood smears and examinations for skin ectoparasites, all of which may be carried out without the need for specialist equipment. More complex techniques – serological methods such enzyme-linked immunosorbent assay (ELISA), immunofluoresence antibody tests (IFAT) and polymerase chain reaction (PCR), for example, are normally referred to external laboratories as they require technical expertise, expensive reagents and equipment. Some important tests for vector-borne pathogens are summarized here, particularly those relating to pets travelling on the European continent, and tests for emergent infections such as lungworms of dogs and cats are described.

Faecal Analysis

How are samples best acquired and stored?

Faecal sample collection, storage and transportation are all important considerations. Only fresh samples should be examined, and tests done as soon as possible. This is because worm eggs will start to develop quickly at room temperature; and if the sample is left for a day or two, a larva may develop inside the egg. This will happen with hookworm eggs, for example, and in some cases the larvae can even hatch out. This is something the veterinary nurse must be aware of since larvated eggs like this may be confused with eggs of *Strongyloides* (a nematode of young animals) which already contain a larva when passed by the host (Fig. 8.1a). Furthermore, samples for submission should not be allowed to come into contact with the ground, and with soil in particular, as environmental free-living larvae, notably those of ascarids, quickly invade faeces, thus complicating diagnosis. The samples

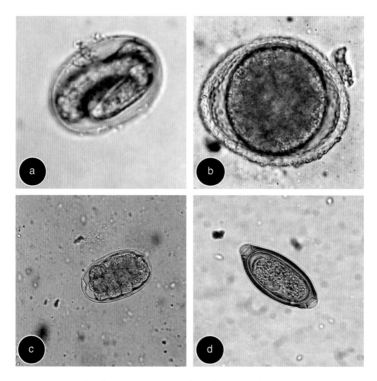

Fig. 8.1. (a) *Strongyloides* spp. egg, produced by female worms as a larvated egg. (b) *Toxocara canis* egg, roughly circular in shape, light brown and with a thick, pitted protein coat. (c) *Uncinaria stenocephala* egg. It has a thin shell and contains an 8–16-cell morula. Some can larvate as they are passed in the faeces. (d) *Trichuris vulpis* egg with its characteristic thick shell and bipolar plugs.

should be stored in secure, leak-proof containers and, if testing is not possible immediately, samples should be placed in the refrigerator.

What is the purpose of a wet faecal smear?

In situations of heavy patent infection, the eggs of gut roundworms, hookworms and tapeworms (e.g. *Toxocara* (Fig. 8.1b), *Uncinaria* (Fig. 8.1c), *Ancylostoma*, *Trichuris* (Fig. 8.1d), *Taenia*, *Echinococcus*), lungworm larvae (*Angiostrongylus* and *Crenosoma* of dogs, and *Aelurostronglyus* of cats) and coccidial infections (*Isospora*) can be detected through microscopic examination of wet smears of faecal samples. A wet smear may be quickly made by mixing and diluting a small amount of the sample in physiological saline, placing a drop on a microscope slide with a coverslip on top and screening at ×100 magnification using a compound microscope. Wet smears can be insensitive in situations other than heavy infections; repeat smears are advisable but interpretation of a negative result must be in context, as for example, parasite eggs can shed intermittently, or in low numbers which cannot be detected without using a concentration method. Cysts of *Giardia intestinalis*, a flagellate protozoan, may also be seen by wet smears but this can be a challenge for the untrained eye, as the cysts (12 μm in size) can be confused with yeasts, for example. Careful examination shows *Giardia* cysts to be rather translucent and pear shaped, with the cyst content divided by a fine longitudinal suture and the content does not entirely fill the cyst on one side.

Can worm eggs be concentrated to improve detection? The bijou method explained

Yes, they can. Most helminth eggs and oocysts (but not *Giardia* and not lungworm larvae) readily float in the saturated salt solutions (e.g. sodium chloride s.g. 1.12; sucrose 1.2) and mixing faecal samples with salts can be used to float up these parasite stages from the faecal mass. The bijou method, for example, uses a small amount of faeces, which is placed inside a 2.5 ml plastic bijou bottle using a wooden stick. The bottle is then three-quarters filled with saturated salt solution and emulsified using the stick. Saturated salt solution is then added drop-wise to the bottle to form a meniscus and a coverslip is immediately placed on top. After 5 min, the coverslip is very quickly removed (with eggs held underneath in the hanging droplet) and placed on a microscope slide; it is screened at ×100 and examined closely at ×400.

Can eggs be quantified? The McMaster technique explained

This method uses the above principle and will detect roundworm and tapeworm eggs, but it is a quantification method (to give an idea of the intensity of infection) and uses a known (weighed out) amount of faeces: 1 g of faeces are weighed and shaken up in 14 ml of saturated salt solution, using a wooden stick to break up the faeces. The mixture is filtered through the strainer into a beaker to remove lumps and the filtered salt solution is thoroughly mixed while taking a sample of the liquid using a Pasteur pipette. One side of the McMaster chamber (Fig. 8.2) is quickly filled. A further sample is taken while swirling the mixture to fill the other chamber. The slide must be left for a few minutes, so that eggs present in the sample have time to float up in the salt solution. The eggs within the ruled area on both sides of the slide are counted and the number of eggs per gram is calculated as follows: 1 g of faeces has been homogenized in 14 ml; the total volume is 15 ml; the volume under one side of the ruled area is 0.15 ml; therefore the number counted on one side must be multiplied by 100 to obtain the number of eggs per gram. It is more accurate to count the eggs in both sides, average the count and then multiply by 100.

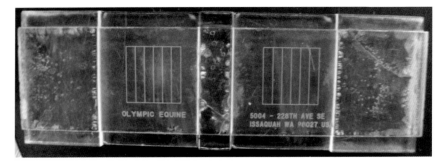

Fig. 8.2. McMaster worm egg-counting slide. The two counting chambers enable the user to count worm eggs in a known volume of faecal suspension (2 × 0.15 ml).

What is the FLOTAC method?

A quantitative flotation method known as the mini-FLOTAC system has been designed to increase sensitivity of faecal flotation. The technique is able not only to diagnosis nematode eggs and coccidian oocysts but also to reveal the presence of lungworm larvae, depending on the faecal solution used. It has also been shown to be more sensitive for eggs and oocysts compared with simple flotation described above.

How can lungworms of dogs and cats be detected in faeces?

There is an increasing prevalence of dog lungworms (*Angiostrongylus vasorum*) in the UK and Europe and parts of the USA. Flotation in salt solution cannot be used to detect the first-stage larvae in faeces and making wet smears may be insensitive. The Baermann method for larval recovery from faeces is a simple and reliable concentration/sedimentation technique, which can be done in practice (Fig. 8.3a).

The method allows diagnosis and monitoring by sedimentation/concentration of mobile first-stage larvae from faeces (Fig. 8.3b). The equipment can be constructed in practice and consists of a plastic funnel with a clipped tube attached. A milk filter lines the inside of the funnel. Water is placed in the funnel and an amount of faeces is then mixed in and allowed to settle overnight. Live first-stage lungworm larvae will migrate out of the faeces and gravitate to the bottom of the tube, which is secured with a clip; a small drop can be examined on a microscope slide. This method is unsuitable for stored samples.

Some laboratories suspend the faecal matter in concentrated zinc sulphate and then centrifuge, thus concentrating lungworm larvae, which are forced to float rapidly to the surface and are then sampled. This salt solution will rapidly distort larvae, however, and examinations have to be made very quickly. Even then, identification of the larvae is impaired.

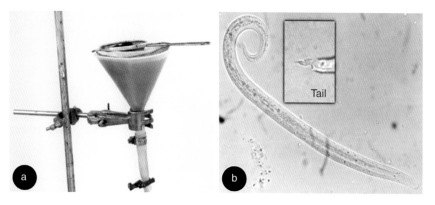

Fig. 8.3. (**a**) Baermann apparatus, for isolation of nematode larvae from faecal materials. (**b**) *Angiostrongylus vasorum* larvae recovered from faeces using Baermann method.

How can faecal smears be stained for Cryptosporidium?

Faecal smears are made from the deposit of a formol-ether stool concentration and allowed to dry for a minimum of 3 h. Smears are fixed in methanol for 3 min, air dried and stained with concentrated carbol-fuchsin for 20 min. The slides are placed in a trough and rinsed in running tap water for 2 min. They are then treated with 1% acid alcohol for a few seconds, changing solution as necessary until the specimen is decolourized (or remains a very pale pink). The slides are rinsed with running tap water in the trough for 2 min, and then counter-stained with malachite green or methylene blue for 30 s. Finally, the slides are rinsed with tap water for 2 min, air dried and mounted with a coverslip, using immersion oil or DPX. Oocysts are examined using ×100 and ×400 objectives. *Cryptosporidium* oocysts (4–6 µm) appear as red oval/round bodies, often stained more densely around the periphery.

Serological Analysis

What is serology and which parasites is it used for?

Basic serology is the immunological detection of circulating parasite antigens or host antibodies to the parasite in body fluids, usually blood, plasma or serum. Serological tests (ELISA, IFAT) involve the serial dilution of the serum or plasma and finding the 'titre' – the most diluted sample that still remains positive (the colour change in the case of an ELISA, and fluorescence in the case of an IFAT). In this way the infection can be quantified.

Serological techniques for diagnosis of dogs and cat parasites in the UK and Europe currently include an ELISA for antigens of *Dirofilaria immitis* and *Angiostrongylus vasorum* and an antibody capture ELISA for *Leishmania* spp. IFATs for various pathogens are also commercially available; for example, for *Anaplasma phagocytophilum* and *Ehrlichia canis*. There has been an increase in point-of-use rapid test systems based on diffusion/chromatography. 'Pet-side' strips are available for *Giardia*, *Cryptosporidium* and *Borrelia burgdorferi*. Diagnostic laboratories offer this type of screening, which particularly important in pets returning from Europe (UK PETS scheme).

Antibody titres are used to provide the infection status (acute or chronic) and to follow the response to treatment. It is important to understand the limitations of these tests. For example, circulating antibodies and antigens may persist after successful elimination of a pathogen, giving a false positive. Serological results can also be affected by antigen or antibody cross-reactions and it is vital to know the published specificity (and sensitivity) of the test. PCR is an assay that can detect very small amounts of parasite DNA and is more sensitive and specific than serological assays.

Molecular Analysis

What is PCR?

In general PCR is not yet commercially available to veterinary practices but is used routinely in research studies. PCR can be used both for the diagnosis of disease and for monitoring dogs undergoing treatment, e.g. for canine leishmaniosis. PCR amplifies DNA from samples. The basic process involves five basic components: the DNA that is to be copied; primers; DNA nucleotide bases; polymerase enzyme; and a buffer. The process involves three steps: denaturing, where the DNA is heated to separate the two strands; annealing, where the temperature is lowered to allow primers to attach; and extending, where the temperature is increased to allow polymerase enzyme to create the new strands of DNA. PCR, carried out only in specialized laboratories, is becoming an increasingly popular and powerful laboratory method for the diagnosis of many diseases. It is sensitive and specific and can assist the practitioner in diagnosing active infection when clinical signs are suspect. It is especially indicated for vector-borne pathogens. PCR can be carried out on most tissues but blood and lymph are the most frequent samples. Tests are available for *Anaplasma, Ehrlichia, Babesia* and *Bartonella*, and *Leishmania*.

Diagnosis of Blood and Tissue Parasite Infection

How are blood films and tissue aspirates stained for parasites?

Giemsa and Leishman's stain are routinely used in parasitology to stain parasites in blood and tissues. The RNA of the parasite stains red and the cytoplasm stains blue. For *Babesia* in red blood cells, a typical staining protocol involves making a thin blood smear and placing it on a staining rack over the sink to flood it with methanol for 30 s. The methanol is tipped off and the slide is air dried. Using a plastic pipette, the smear is covered with Giemsa stain (diluted 1:10) and left in the diluted stain for 15 min. The stain is carefully rinsed off with tap water into a waste pot and left to dry. A drop of immersion oil is placed on the dry blood smear and the stained smear is examined using the oil immersion lens.

Diagnosis of Ectoparasite Infestation

What about ectoparasites? How can skin be examined for mange mites and other arthropods?

Examination of skin and tissue may reveal all the life cycle stages of an ectoparasite, including eggs, larvae, nymph and adult stages and moulted cuticles. Examination of old lesions may reveal dead and degenerated ecto- parasites or parts of these. For surface-feeding non-burrowing mites (e.g. *Cheyletiella*), repeat samples should be obtained by gently scraping the skin and examining scales, hairs and debris on a microscope slide in saline, and with a coverslip placed on top. The scrapings can also be examined dry, under the high power of a dissecting stereo microscope, whereby moving mites can be seen against a dark background, particularly when particles of debris have adhered to the mite's body hairs.

Deeper skin scrapings using a scalpel blade (with a little liquid paraffin added) are necessary to recover burrowing mites such as *Sarcoptes* and *Demodex*. In severe mange, often where scab material is present, removed tissue can be macerated in 10% potassium hydroxide for 10 min; the re- sulting fluid is placed on a microscope slide with a coverslip and examined under low power (×100). Higher magnification is needed to see *Demodex* mites. There is an ELISA available for the detection of *Sarcoptes scabiei*. The presence of fleas can be confirmed by brushing dirt and debris from the ani- mal's coat on to a piece of filter paper or similar absorbent substrate. When a small drop of water is added, the material will turn bright red. The blood is excess host blood excreted by the flea.

It is sometimes important to identify arthropods, e.g. to determine the spe- cies of flea that is biting an animal, when monitoring a control programme. This is best done by making a semi-permanent preparation. Soft-bodied arthropods (including mange mites) may be processed by placing them dir- ectly into lactophenol or Berlese fluid on a microscope slide with a coverslip. To make good preparations for identification of hard-bodied mites (such as *Dermanyssus gallinae*) and fleas, a processing step is needed. This is because the latter have dark chitinous cuticles and may also have ingested blood, so clearing the cuticle is necessary by incubation in 10% potassium hydroxide followed by washing and dehydration in a series of alcohols. The specimen is then placed in xylene and mounted on a glass slide using a resinous mountant (DPX or similar).

Self-Assessment Questions

1. **How are parasites in blood cells detected?**

    (a) By staining with Giemsa

    (b) By examining a wet smear

    (c) By lysing the blood

    (d) By concentrating the blood cells

2. **How does a PCR work?**

    (a) By detecting parasite antibodies

    (b) By detecting parasite antigens

    (c) By amplifying parasite DNA

    (d) By amplifying both host DNA and the parasite DNA

3. **The McMaster method is for which of the following?**

    (a) Quantifying worm eggs in faecal samples

    (b) Detecting antigens

    (c) Detecting antibodies

    (d) Detecting *cryptosporidium* oocysts

4. **Mange mites are best detected by which of the following?**

    (a) McMaster counting slide

    (b) The bijou bottle method

    (c) IFAT

    (d) Skin scrapings

5. **The gold standard method for detection of lungworms is which of the following?**

    (a) The Baermann technique

    (b) Detecting antibodies using ELISA

    (c) Transtracheal wash

    (d) Larval faecal culture

9 Parasite Control Clinics

What is the role of veterinary nurses in parasite control clinics?

Veterinary nurses play a vital role in the education of clients on parasite control. Many clients feel more comfortable discussing parasite prevention with a nurse as they are often perceived to be more approachable and available to the client for longer periods of time. Opportunities to discuss parasite control may occur in dedicated parasite clinics, at reception or in telephone conversations. Through these varieties of medium, nurses can form bonds with clients and, by gathering information about their lifestyles, can assess parasite risk and maximize preventive treatment compliance. As well as recording information, assessing risk and giving advice, nurses may also perform parasite diagnostic tests, such as coat tape strippings, flea combing, skin scrapes, urinalysis, blood smear examination, serology and faecal flotation.

Whether a practice has one dedicated parasite nurse or several will depend on the size of the practice and nurse availability. If multiple nurses are involved, it is vital that advice and protocols are consistent and that parasite knowledge is kept up to date.

What information should be obtained from clients in parasite control clinics?

The client should be asked questions that allow a comprehensive picture of parasite risk to be established, but also to establish lifestyle factors that will influence treatment efficacy and compliance. These will vary from country to country and the parasites that are endemic there, but examples are as follows.

What is the client's current parasite control plan? The client may already be using anti-parasitic treatments, so it is important to find out what these are and the frequency being administered, to establish if they are sufficient for the pet's needs.

Has the pet had any previous perceived or confirmed reactions to treatment? Certain products may need to be avoided due to drug reactions. These may be common mild side effects, such as vomiting after administration of an oral product or localized skin reaction after administration of a spot-on solution. While not serious, these reactions are likely to reduce compliance and be debilitating over time. More serious reactions, such as anaphylaxis, will mean that products cannot be used, but even adverse events that have not been confirmed to be due to the parasite treatment given will reduce future compliance if the owner perceives a link between the two.

Does the client have a preference for a specific treatment formulation? Compliance is likely to be increased if the owner has a strong preference for a tablet, spot-on solution or collar.

Is the pet washed with shampoo or does the pet frequently swim? The efficacy of products that are absorbed into the sebum layer, such as fipronil and imidacloprid, can be affected by shampoos and frequent or prolonged swimming.

Does the pet eat a raw unprocessed diet, scavenge or hunt? Eating a raw unprocessed diet, scavenging and/or hunting increases the risk of both tapeworm and *Toxocara* spp. infection.

Does the pet come into regular contact with young children or immune-suppressed adults? These are high-risk groups for human toxocariasis and cats and dogs in regular contact with them should be treated monthly for *Toxocara* infection to minimize risk.

Does the pet visit areas of tall grass or bracken? The risk of ticks and tick-borne diseases is increased, particularly if the land is shared with domestic ruminants or deer.

Does the pet have a history of previous tick exposure? If the lifestyle of the pet has exposed it to ticks in the past, it is likely to occur again in the future.

Do pet dogs eat slugs and snails or regularly consume grass? The accidental or deliberate consumption of slugs and snails will potentially expose pet dogs to *Angiostrongylus vasorum* infection (Fig. 9.1).

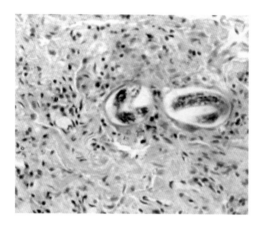

Fig. 9.1. Histopathology of dog lung tissue showing *Angiostrongylus vasorum* larvae associated with inflammatory reaction.

Active listening

Methods such as active listening are useful in reinforcing information from the client. This method consists of the veterinary nurse asking a question and then repeating the client's answer back to them to ensure the meaning has been understood. In doing so, the nurse can confirm the information originally given but also allow the client to expand on their answer.

How can the nurse help to improve owner compliance?

A variety of methods are available to explain the need for parasite control and how to implement a parasite control programme. Often, using a variety of techniques helps to reinforce messages and improve compliance. Information on how to use parasiticides and the frequency of application needs to be conveyed, as well as simple practical techniques such as how to use a tick hook. Different techniques include:

- talking to the client directly;
- using diagrams and videos to demonstrate life cycles and techniques;
- demonstrating administration of parasiticides;
- asking clients to practise administering parasiticides in the clinic to see if they are being applied correctly;
- giving the opportunity for the client to practise with spot-on pipettes and tablets containing no active ingredient; and
- offering written material for the client to take away, such as instructions, frequency reminders, parasite information and life cycle charts.

The role of the veterinary nurse should continue after initial advice has been given by regularly contacting the client to ensure that lifestyle circumstances have not changed and that compliance is still being achieved.

Should the nurse clinically examine the patient in nurse clinics?

A full clinical examination should take place in nurse-run clinics and if any abnormalities are detected, the patient can be passed on to a veterinary surgeon. Simple clinical information can be established such as the presence of fleas and ticks, body condition score, coat quality, heart and respiratory rate and body temperature. The patient's weight should also be recorded for accurate treatment dosing.

Empowering nurses to deliver evidence-based service

In order for veterinary nurses to be able to speak knowledgeably and in lay terminology to clients about strategic deworming programmes, they must first have knowledge of worm life cycles, mode of infection, how to decrease exposure, diagnostic testing, consequences of infection and the potential human health risk. Nurses need to be empowered with regular updates on the latest developments in strategic parasite control guidelines. By offering a comprehensive training programme, including formal teaching (Fig. 9.2), nurses will gain confidence in dealing with informed clients and so can easily address questions raised by clients about parasite control.

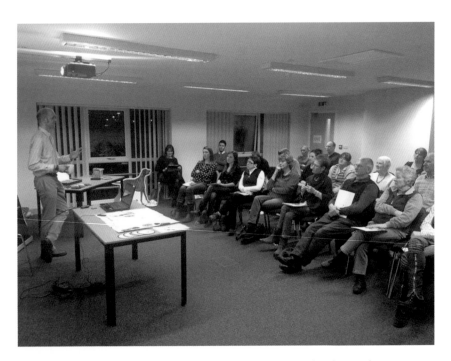

Fig. 9.2. Training event about effective means of parasite control in dogs and cats.

Self-Assessment Questions

1. **How often should dogs living with children be treated for** *Toxocara* **roundworm infection?**

   (a) Monthly

   (b) Every 3 months

   (c) Every 6 months

   (d) Annually

2. **Slug consumption by dogs is a risk factor for which parasite?**

   (a) *Angiostrongylus vasorum*

   (b) *Toxocara canis*

   (c) *Taenia ovis*

   (d) *Echinococcus granulosus*

3. **Long grass and bracken are risk factors for which of the following parasites?**

   (a) *Leishmania infantum*

   (b) Tapeworm

   (c) Heartworm

   (d) Ticks

4. **Unprocessed raw meat consumption is a risk factor for which of the following parasites?**

   (a) *Leishmania infantum*

   (b) Tapeworm

   (c) Heartworm

   (d) Ticks

5. **Hunting/predation is a risk factor for which of the following parasites?**

   (a) *Leishmania infantum*

   (b) Tapeworm

   (c) Ticks

   (d) Heartworm

10 Parasite Control and Pet Travel

How do pet travel and importation affect parasite distributions?

Pet travel and pet importation are increasing in most European countries and North America year on year. The UK, for example, saw an increase in travelling dogs from 140,000 in 2012 to 164,800 in 2015. Similarly, the numbers of dogs being imported into the UK for commercial purposes increased from 26,399 in 2014 to 28,344 in 2015. This increase in pet travel has occurred at a time of increased human migration and climate change, providing favourable conditions for the rapid spread of parasitic diseases and their vectors. This, in turn, increases the risk of pets and their owners encountering exotic agents while abroad and bringing them back to their country of residence. Imported animals may also be carrying non-native pathogens and vectors. These factors can increase the risk of introduction of parasites in a number of different ways. Veterinary nurses must therefore be aware of exotic parasites being present in imported and travelled pets.

Introduction of parasites into existing vector populations ('vectors waiting for a disease') *Dermacentor reticulatus* and *Ixodes* spp. ticks are vectors of *Babesia canis* and tick-borne encephalitis (TBE), respectively. Many countries have long-established populations of these vectors but are not endemic for *B. canis* or TBE. If these vector-borne agents were introduced to these countries, they would be able to infect existing vector populations.

Introduction of parasites into areas where new vectors have established *Thelazia callipaeda* has spread northwards across Europe in the wake of its *Phortica* spp. fruit fly vector. While climate, vehicle transport and wind dispersal are factors in the distribution of the fruit fly, pet movements introduce infected animals into areas where the fruit fly is already present.

© CAB International 2018. *Parasites and Pets* (Elsheikha, Wright & McGarry)

Introduction of vectors and parasites together *Dermacentor* ticks infected with *B. canis* and *Rhipicephalus* ticks infected with *Ehrlichia canis* have moved southwards and northwards, respectively, through Europe. As the ticks have expanded their distribution, the parasites they transmit have moved with them, increasing their endemic range.

Introduction of vector-borne parasites that are then transmitted in the absence of the vector *Leishmania infantum* has established in countries with no sandfly vector, such as Canada, purely through venereal transmission.

How can the risk of travelling pets being infected with exotic parasites be minimized?

A cohesive strategy is required to keep travelling pets and their owners safe while maintaining biosecurity. This is achieved through consistent accurate advice to clients regarding protection against parasites endemic in the countries to be visited. Preventive steps include the following:

Preventive treatments while abroad Pets travelling to heartworm-endemic countries should be placed on a macrocyclic lactone while abroad, starting before travel and continuing for at least one treatment after return. Pets should be on a tick preventive, which should also be a licensed fly repellent treatment if travelling to a country endemic for leishmaniosis. This treatment should be started a week before travel and continued on return. A *Leishmania* vaccine is also available for dogs. Dogs travelling to *Echinococcus* spp. endemic countries should be treated monthly with praziquantel to prevent patent infection establishing, which would put owners at immediate zoonotic risk.

Avoiding fly bites In addition to the use of fly repellents, the use of pyrethroid-impregnated bed nets, sleeping upstairs or camping in breezy locations will also help to reduce numbers of fly bites. This should be used as an adjunct to other treatments in heartworm and *Leishmania* endemic countries, rather than alternatives.

Checking for ticks and removing them at least every 24 h Owners checking themselves and their pets for ticks every 24 h and removing any found (Fig. 10.1a) with a tick hook will help to reduce tick-borne disease exposure. This is important even if a tick preventive product is being used, as while they are highly efficacious in reducing tick-borne disease exposure, none is 100% effective.

What precautionary measures should be taken for imported pets?

The risk of imported pets introducing novel parasites and vectors can be mitigated by employing a number of measures.

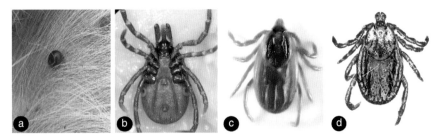

Fig. 10.1. (**a**) Adult *Ixodes ricinus* (the sheep tick, wood tick, deer tick or castor bean tick) attached to the hair of the host. This tick is found mainly in areas of rough grazing, moorland, woodland and areas where wild deer and rabbit are in abundance. (**b**) Ventral view of *Ixodes ricinus* tick. (**c**) Dorsal view of *Rhipicephalus sanguineus* (the brown dog tick, kennel tick). (**d**) Dorsal view of *Dermacentor reticulatus* (the ornate cow tick or marsh tick), the vector of *Babesia canis*. (Courtesy of Professor Richard Wall, Bristol University, UK.)

Treating imported dogs with praziquantel   If dogs are being imported into a country free from *Echinococcus granulosus* or *Echinococcus multilocularis* infection, treatment with praziquantel on arrival will eliminate any patent infection the dogs may be carrying.

Checking pets for ticks   Checking for ticks and identifying them on imported pets (Fig. 10.1b,c,d) is vital to prevent exotic ticks and tick-borne diseases from establishing endemic foci, but also in establishing which potential tick-borne diseases the pet may have been exposed to.

Being aware of relevant clinical signs in imported pets   Clinical signs in imported pets should be cross-checked against parasitic diseases endemic in the country of origin.

Screening for exotic disease   Imported pets should be screened for *Leishmania*, heartworm and tick-borne diseases so that if clinical disease develops it can be detected early and exposure to endemic vectors can be limited.

What is the role of nurses in pet travel clinics?

The veterinary nurse plays a vital role in delivering the services described in practice and maintaining both national biosecurity and individual pet health as a result. Veterinary nurses are often the first point of call for pet owners visiting the practice, whether for routine check-ups, pet travel advice or veterinary diagnosis. They are therefore likely to be at the forefront of recognizing relevant clinical signs in newly imported pets, carrying out diagnostic tests, communicating risks and compliance with pet owners. Veterinary nurses are essential in the following:

Pet travel clinics   Many practices offer a pet travel clinic led by a veterinary nurse for travelling pets. These offer an initial assessment of the risks and requirements when travelling abroad and are the first step in creating tailored parasite control plans for the pet before, during and after travel.

Recording of cases   The job of recording exotic vectors or disease cases often falls to the veterinary nurse. It is an essential service to monitor disease and contribute to national and international disease surveillance.

Recognizing exotic disease cases   Veterinary nurses must be prepared for a variety of parasitic diseases to be presented to veterinary practices in travelled and imported pets. Not only should veterinary nurses remain vigilant for clinical signs in travelled and imported pets that may be exotic in origin, but they should also be aware of the risk of subclinical carriers. Nurses play an important role in conveying these risks and encouraging screening and compliance, especially to new owners of imported pets.

Self-Assessment Questions

1. **Which of the following is a vector for *Babesia canis*?**

    (a) *Dermacentor reticulatus*

    (b) Culicine mosquitoes

    (c) *Phortica* spp. fruit flies

    (d) Sandflies

2. **Which of the following is a vector for *Thelazia callipaeda* eye worm?**

    (a) *Dermacentor reticulatus*

    (b) Culicine mosquitoes

    (c) *Phortica* spp. fruit flies

    (d) Sandflies

3. **Which of the following is a treatment for *Echinococcus multilocularis* tapeworm?**

    (a) Fenbendazole

    (b) Ivermectin

    (c) Permethrin

    (d) Praziquantel

4. **How soon should a licensed fly repellent be administered to a dog before travelling to a *Leishmania* endemic country?**

   (a) 1 day

   (b) 2 days

   (c) 1 week

   (d) 2 weeks

5. **In the absence of its vector, how has *Leishmania* established endemic foci in some countries?**

   (a) By switching vectors

   (b) Through dog bites

   (c) By airborne transmission

   (d) By venereal transmission

Glossary

The purpose of this glossary is to include terms mentioned in the book; as well as key terms that do not appear in the text, but may be useful for further understanding of the subject. The glossary is not a definitive list of the terminology used in veterinary parasitology.

anaphylaxis: A strong hypersensitivity reaction in which the individual may collapse, stop breathing and die

anthelmintic: A chemical drug used to remove worms, usually from the intestinal tract of a host

antibody: Serum protein (immunoglobulin) synthesized by lymphoid cells in response to an antigenic stimulus

antigen: Any substance that can stimulate an immune response

basis capituli: Pseudo-head of a tick; bears the mouthparts and the probing and sensory structures

bradyzoite: Slow-growing zoite or meront of the pseudocyst of *Toxoplasma* and related cyst-forming coccidian protozoa

buccal capsule: Mouth cavity of a nematode

bursa (copulatory bursa): A cuticular copulatory structure at the posterior end of males of the order Strongylida. It is useful in nematode taxonomy and species identification

cellular immunity: A specific response to an antigen in which lymphoid cells are the primary effectors

cercaria (-iae): A free-living larval trematode that develops from a sporocyst or redia in snail intermediate hosts

chemokines: Small proteins that attract and stimulate cells of the immune defence; produced by many cells in response to infection.

commensal: A form of symbiosis between two organisms where one derives benefit, whereas the other is unaffected

control: General term comprising therapy and prevention (prophylaxis)

convalescence period: The time that follows the disappearance of clinical symptoms until the complete throw-off of the parasite

coprophagous: Feeding on faecal material

cuticle: A secreted surface covering that is generally considered to be non-living

cyst: A general term used when an organism has a membrane surrounding it, whether the covering is of its own making or of host origin. Cystic stage is a common resistant stage in some protozoa

cytokines: Soluble proteins produced by cells in response to various stimuli, including parasitic infection; they affect the behaviour of other cells both locally and at a distance, by binding to specific cytokine receptors

definitive host: A primary host, in which a parasite is able to reach maturity, i.e. its adult sexual form, and where sexual reproduction takes place

dioecious: Separate sexes

ectoparasite: A parasite that lives on the external surface or in the integument of a host

egg: The germ cell of a female; an ovum

emerging parasite: A parasite population responsible for a marked increase in disease incidence, usually as result of changed societal, environmental or population factors

endemic: A disease or disease agent that is present continually in a region or among a certain group of animals

engorgement: Distension of a feeding tick or fly with blood; cannot occur in male hard ticks, because their back is covered completely by a hard scutum

enzootic: A disease or disease agent that occurs in an animal population at all times

epidemic: A disease or disease agent that spreads rapidly through a population

epidemiology: The study of the causes of disease; the complex of factors that lead to disease outbreaks

epizootic: A disease or disease agent that spreads rapidly through an animal population

feral: Wild; a feral cycle of a parasitic agent is one that takes place in the wild as opposed to an urban site

festoon: Raised areas separated by grooves, situated around the posterior margin of the cuticle of hard ticks of certain species

fomites: Inanimate objects that may be contaminated with microorganisms and become vehicles for the transmission of infectious agents

gamogony (= gametogony): Formation of gametes

granuloma:	A swelling composed of leucocytes, fluid and connective tissue; often a foreign-body reaction
haematophagous:	Blood-sucking; usually refers to the feeding habits of various insects and acarines such as mosquitoes and ticks
haematuria:	Blood in the urine; a condition seen in some individuals infected with blood parasites, e.g. *Plasmodium falciparum*
haemorrhage:	Escape of blood from vessels
hermaphroditism:	The presence of both male and female reproductive organs in the same organism that is capable of reproducing on its own
heterogenic:	Reproduction in which sexual and asexual generations alternate, as in the nematode *Strongyloides*
heteroxenous:	Having more than one host required to complete a life cycle, such as in the digenetic trematodes
hexacanth:	The motile, six-hooked, first-stage larva of certain tapeworms; stage that hatches from the cestode egg and infects the intermediate host
homoxenous:	A parasite that has a direct life cycle or one in which only a single host is required for its completion
horizontal transmission:	Transmission of a parasitic agent among members of a group
host range:	The number of species of hosts that can be infected by a parasitic agent
humoral immunity:	A specific response to an antigen in which the principal effectors are antibodies that circulate in the blood
hyperaemia:	An abnormally large amount of blood in a tissue
hyperplasia:	An abnormally high number of cells in a tissue
hypersensitivity (= *allergy*):	A condition in which a mammal is sensitized to a particular substance and has an abnormally strong reaction when the substance is encountered again
hypertrophy:	An abnormal increase in the size of a tissue or an organ
immune memory:	A property provided by specialized B and T lymphocytes (memory B and T cells) that respond rapidly on re-exposure to the parasitic infection that originally induced them
immunity:	A specific response in vertebrates to a foreign protein in which cells respond by producing humoral and/or cellular antibodies
immunopathology:	Pathological changes partly or completely caused by the immune response
incubation period:	The period beginning from the time of an infection until the onset of clinical signs; usually longer than the prepatent period

inflammation: A general term for the complex response by a vertebrate to physical, chemical, or biological insult that gives rise to local accumulation of white blood cells and fluid; characterized by pain, reddening, increased temperature and swelling at the site

innate response: The first line of defence; able to function continually in the host without prior exposure to the invading parasite. This complex system comprises, in part, cytokines, sentinel cells, complement and natural killer cells

integrated control: The use of several measures to control different parasites or parasite stages present on the animal and stages present in the environment

intermediate host: A host in or on which a pathogen spends a part of its life cycle, but does not reach sexual maturity

juvenile: An organism that is similar to the adult of the species but is sexually immature

killed vaccine: A vaccine made by taking an authentic disease-causing parasite and treating it with chemicals to reduce infectivity to non-detectable level

larva: An embryo that becomes self-sustaining and independent before it has developed the characteristic features of the adult form

live attenuated vaccine: A vaccine made from parasitic mutants that have reduced virulence and lack the capacity to cause a disease

memory cells: A subset of B and T lymphocytes maintained after each encounter with a foreign antigen; they survive for years and are ready to respond and proliferate upon subsequent encounter with the same antigen

merozoite: Product of merogony; usually an elongate organism that infects another host cell to undergo either merogony again or gamogony

metacercaria (-iae): The infective stage of a fluke enclosed in a protective cyst that resists adverse environmental conditions. This stage develops from the cercaria and is infective for the definitive host

metacestode: Immature tapeworm ('larval' cestode) that develops from the hexacanth embryo (oncosphere) and grows in the intermediate host (mammal), but one not yet sexually mature

microfilaria (-iae): First-stage larva of a filarial worm transmitted to the biting insect from the definitive host

monoclonal antibody: An antibody of a single specificity made by a clone of antibody-producing cells

monoecious: Both male and female sex organs in one individual; hermaphroditic

moulting (= *ecdysis*):	Shedding of an external covering such as integument or exoskeleton; in arthropods and nematodes, shedding the external covering allows the parasite to expand in its new skin
mucosal immunity:	Immune responses expressed at mucosal surfaces
mucous membrane:	Any of several moist surfaces in the body of vertebrates in which there are mucus-secreting or goblet cells; examples are the orbit of the eye, nasal passages, inside the mouth
mutualism (*mutualist*):	A form of symbiosis between two organisms in which both benefit from the relationship
myiasis:	Invasion of healthy body tissues by the larvae of flies
nymph:	The pre-adult stage of an insect, or acarine which has hemimetabolic development in a terrestrial environment
occult infection:	Hidden infection; one in which no eggs or larvae are produced. For example, infections can be occult when only worms of one sex are present of a species that requires mating to produce eggs or larvae
oedema:	Abnormal accumulation of fluid in cells, tissues, or tissue spaces resulting in swelling
oocyst:	A stage in the life cycle of certain members of the phylum Apicomplexa in which the zygote secretes a wall around itself; often highly resistant to environmental conditions
operculum:	Lid or cap-like structure at one or both ends of certain worm eggs, e.g. *Trichuris* and fluke; the larval parasite emerges from the egg at the operculum
opportunistic:	A potential pathogen that typically does not cause disease in a healthy host, but can in particular situations cause disease; for example, owing to the compromised immune system of the host.
ornate:	Coloured; patterned (cf. inornate tick)
ovum (*-a*):	The female germ cell
parasite pathogenesis:	The process by which parasitic infections cause disease; the progression of a disease
parasitic (*parasite*):.	A non-mutual symbiosis between two species where one, the parasite, benefits at the expense of the other, the host. Parasites do not kill their hosts but exploit them for resources necessary for their survival. Obligate parasites cannot complete their life cycles and reproduce without a suitable host
paratenic host:	An atypical (alternative) intermediate host that harbours the stage infective for the definitive host, which remains active and unchanged. If a suitable definitive host ingests the paratenic host or a part of it containing the infective stage, the parasite can grow to maturity

parthenogenesis: The laying of fertile eggs by a female without the need for fertilization by a male. It is common in some nematodes, such as *Strongyloides*

passive immunization: Direct administration of the products of the immune response (e.g. antibodies or stimulated immune cells) obtained from appropriate donor(s) to a patient

patent period: The period during which the parasite can be detected by diagnostic laboratory methods

pathogenic (pathogen): A broad term that refers to the ability of an organism to cause disease.

pathogenicity: The ability of a pathogen to overcome host defences and cause disease

period of relapse: The period during which the symptoms reappear without reinfection

period of symptoms: The period during which the disease symptoms could be clinically recognized, such as high temperature, diarrhea, coughing, etc.

persistent infection: An infection that is not cleared by the combined actions of the innate and acquired immune response

plasma: The fluid portion of the blood

prepatent period: The period that begins from the time of infection with the infective stage until the appearance of diagnostic stages such as eggs, larvae and cysts

prevalence: The proportion of a defined population affected by a disease at a particular point in time

prevention: Measures taken prior to any infection/infestation of the animal with parasites, to prevent the establishment of an infection/infestation

primary antibody response: The initial response of B cells when first exposed to an infection

proglottid: A body segment of a tapeworm containing a complete set of reproductive organs

pro-inflammatory cytokines: Cytokines produced predominantly by activated immune cells; responsible for amplification of inflammatory reactions

prophylaxis: Measures carried out to prevent the transmission of the parasitic agent or the occurrence of disease

quarantine: Restriction in the freedom of movement of humans or animals in order to contain the spread of any infectious or contagious disease; the length of time is slightly longer than the longest known incubation period of the disease in question

repellent: Compound that makes a host unattractive to an ectoparasite and thus can prevent attack or establishment

reportable disease: A disease that, by law, must be reported to a health authority. In general, such diseases are of special concern to the health of the human or animal population; examples are malaria, foot-and-mouth disease and tuberculosis

reservoir: The habitat or host that harbours an infectious agent, where it can live, grow and multiply

scolex: The holdfast or organ by which a tapeworm attaches to the intestine of its host

scutum: A hard plate or shield on the dorsum behind the capitulum of hard ticks. The scutum is much more extensive in male ticks than in females

secondary antibody response: The antibody response produced after a subsequent infection with the same antigen or parasite

serum: The fluid part of vertebrate blood after the fibrin has been removed

sign: Any objective evidence of disease, e.g. fever, diarrhoea, or skin rash

strobila: A chain of tapeworm proglottids or segments

sylvatic: Refers to forest or a wooded area; used as an adjective to describe the location of a disease cycle in the wild

symptomatic treatment: Non-specific therapy of a disease that is designed to reduce the symptoms or the effects

systemic infection: An infection that results in spread to many organs of the body

tachyzoite: Rapidly growing zoite, characteristic of the early stage of infection with *Toxoplasma* and related organisms of the phylum Apicomplexa

therapeutic index: Margin of safety of a drug; the difference between the dose that kills parasites and the dose that harms the host

therapy: Any medical intervention to cure a disease; this includes the use of veterinary medicinal products to eliminate an existing parasite infection/infestation

transmission: The passing of an infectious agent from one host to another host. Direct transmission routes include: physical contact, contact with a contaminated environment or surface, airborne transmission and faecal–oral transmission. Indirect transmission routes involve another organism, such as an insect vector or intermediate host

trophozoite: The growing, feeding stage of a protozoan

vaccination: Inoculation of healthy individuals with attenuated or related microorganisms, or their antigenic products, to elicit an immune response that will protect against later infection by the corresponding pathogen

vector: An organism that carries and transmits a pathogen from an infected individual to another individual

vertical transmission: Transmission of a parasite from one generation to the next through the egg or *in utero*

virulence: A property of a pathogen, such as specific structural elements or biochemical compounds commonly called virulence factors that cause damage to the host.

zoonosis: An infectious disease caused by an organism, such as a bacterium, such as a bacterium, virus, parasite or fungus, transmissible between wildlife or domesticated animals and humans. Examples include: (i) the Lyme disease bacterium *Borrelia* transmitted to humans by ticks from a natural reservoir in rodents; and (ii) *Cryptosporidium parvum*, a parasite found in cats, dogs and farmed animals and transmitted as a cyst in contaminated water, food, or through the faecal–oral route

zoonotic agent: An organism that causes a zoonosis

zoonotic potential: The potential for infectious diseases of wildlife or domestic animals to be transmitted to humans

Bibliography

Bowman, D.D. (2013) *Georgis' Parasitology for Veterinarians*, 10th edn. Saunders, St Louis, Missouri.

Conboy, G. (2009) Cestodes of dogs and cats in North America. *Veterinary Clinics of North America. Small Animal Practice* 39(6), 1075–1090.

Despommier, D.D., Griffin, D., Gwadz, R.W., Hotez, P.J. and Knirsch, C. (2017) *Parasitic Diseases*. Parasites Without Borders, Inc., New York.

Elsheikha, H.M. and Khan, N.A. (2010) Protozoa traversal of the blood–brain barrier to invade the central nervous system. *FEMS Microbiology Reviews* 34(4), 532–553.

Elsheikha, H.M. and Khan, N.A. (2011) *Essentials of Veterinary Parasitology*. Caister Academic Press, Wymondham, Norfolk, UK.

Elsheikha, H.M. and Jarroll, E.J. (2017) *Illustrated Dictionary of Parasitology in the Post-Genomic Era*. Caister Academic Press, Wymondham, Norfolk, UK

Elsheikha, H.M. and Patterson, J. (2013). *Self-Assessment Colour Review: Veterinary Parasitology*. Manson Publishing, London.

Jacobs, D., Fox, M., Gibbons, L. and Hermosilla, C. (2015) *Principles of Veterinary Parasitology*. Wiley-Blackwell, Chichester, UK.

Loker, E.S. and Hofkin, B. (2015). *Parasitology: a Conceptual Approach*. Garland Science, Taylor & Francis Group, New York.

Taylor, M., Coop, B. and Wall, R. (2015) *Veterinary Parasitology*. Wiley-Blackwell, Oxford.

Self-assessment Answers

Chapter 1
1. (b)

2. (a)

3. (a)

4. (d)

5. (d)

Chapter 2
1. (a)

2. (d)

3. (a)

4. (b)

5. (a)

Chapter 3
1. (b)

2. (a)

3. (d)

4. (a)

5. (c)

Chapter 4

1. (d)

2. (b)

3. (d)

4. (c)

5. (c)

Chapter 5
Fleas

1. (c)

2. (a)

3. (b)

4. (d)

5. (b)

Lice

1. (b)

2. (d)

3. (c)

4. (d)

5. (a)

Mites

1. (a)

2. (d)

3. (c)

4. (b)

5. (d)

Ticks

1. (d)

2. (a)

3. (b)

4. (a)

5. (d)

Leishmaniosis

1. (c)

2. (d)

3. (b)

4. (a)

5. (c)

Chapter 6

1. (a)

2. (d)

3. (c)

4. (a)

5. (a)

Chapter 7

1. (c)

2. (d)

3. (d)

4. (a)

5. (b)

Chapter 8

1. (a)

2. (c)

3. (a)

4. (d)

5. (a)

Chapter 9

1. (a)

2. (a)

3. (d)

4. (b)

5. (b)

Chapter 10

1. (a)

2. (c)

3. (d)

4. (c)

5. (d)

Index

Page numbers in **bold** type refer to figures and tables.